A Philosophical Handbook for Pain Medicine Practice

Milton Cohen • John Quintner

A Philosophical Handbook for Pain Medicine Practice

Springer

Milton Cohen
Former adjunct professor, St Vincent's Clinical School, University of New South Wales
Retired specialist pain medicine physician, Current independent scholar
Mosman, NSW, Australia

John Quintner
Former consultant, Arthritis and Osteoporosis Foundation of Western Australia
Retired specialist pain medicine physician, Current independent scholar
Mount Claremont, WA, Australia

ISBN 978-981-92-1681-9 ISBN 978-981-92-1682-6 (eBook)
https://doi.org/10.1007/978-981-92-1682-6

This Springer imprint is published by the registered company Springer Nature Singapore Pte Ltd.
The registered company address is: 152 Beach Road, #21-01/04 Gateway East, Singapore 189721, Singapore

This clinical handbook is dedicated to those whose voices may not have been heard and to those who want to hear them.

It would be a great thing to understand Pain in all its meanings.
Peter Mere Latham (1989–1875)
General Remarks on the Practice of Medicine, British Medical Journal 1861

Foreword

In the myth of Ulysses, the hero navigates between Scylla and Charybdis with wax plugs in his ears, resisting the song of the sirens—a song that promises wisdom but leads to destruction. Milton Cohen and John Quintner have undertaken a similar voyage in this book: traversing the most liminal gorges and landscapes of pain's topography without heeding received wisdom, guided by their own judgment and iron determination. Where others succumb to the seductive song of familiar constructs and comfortable explanations, they hold course toward more demanding but more honest waters.

There is a kind of book that is not written to be read comfortably, but to be thought through uncomfortably. *A Philosophical Handbook for Pain Medicine Practice* is one of them. The authors have undertaken a difficult and necessary task: compelling pain medicine to look in the mirror and confront the conceptual imprecisions, misnomers, and logical fallacies that have colonized its discourse for decades.

Indeed, the myth of Ulysses leads us naturally to that of Sisyphus. For too long, pain medicine has melancholically rolled the same stone up the hill again and again—the same debates, the same terminological errors, the same conceptual confusions—only to watch it roll back down and begin anew. This book invites us to something radically different: to stop, release the stone, and push in a different way. Not to exert more effort, but to direct our effort in another direction. Not more repetition, but conceptual evolution.

This handbook is not destructive criticism, but a demand for epistemological discipline. The authors remind us that the language we use is not neutral: it shapes our understanding, guides our interventions, and ultimately affects the patient before us. When we reify pain by treating it as a thing, we are not making minor terminological errors. We are perpetuating confusions that have real clinical consequences—confusions that add unnecessary suffering to real people in pain.

What makes this work singular is its insistence that philosophy is not an academic luxury but a clinical tool. Approaching the nature of pain from a non-substantialist ontology is not an exercise in metaphysics: it has real repercussions for clinical engagement with patients. The integration of Husserl or Bourdieu with daily pain practice is not ornamental: it is the scaffolding that enables the construction of a clinical encounter based on intersubjectivity, mutual validation, and the redistribution of symbolic capital. The authors demonstrate that while nociception is not sufficient, it is necessary for pain to occur, and that understanding this distinction—along with the profound clinical and ethical implications that this truth contains—is not theoretical subtlety but the foundation for a more honest medicine. And honesty, at times, is uncomfortable, for it requires abandoning familiar constructs that have organized our clinical practice for years or decades.

This handbook does not offer recipes. You will not find treatment protocols or clinical algorithms here. What you will find is something more valuable and more difficult: a conceptual map for navigating pain's complexity without deceptive simplifications.

Reading this book demands effort. But effort has its reward: seeing clearly. And seeing clearly, in pain medicine, is the first step—perhaps the most important—toward a more just, more honest, and more humane practice. The authors do not ask us to accept their conclusions blindly, but to think rigorously. In times when medicine tends toward simplification and slogans, this handbook is a reminder that the complexity of pain deserves the complexity of thought.

In Greek myth, the sea was wine-dark. The field of pain often is as well. This book is also a lighthouse amid the darkness, from which Milton and John signal a new course. Dear reader, now that you are about to delve into these lucid pages, close your eyes for a moment and breathe deeply: I invite you to stop, release the stone, and learn to traverse pain's hillside in a different way, far from the sirens' songs. It is my hope that this work inspires you to see your patients in a renewed way, encourages you to revisit many concepts in the field that you had taken for granted, to have difficult conversations and to pose honest debates. But above all, I would like to tell you that Milton and John's is a lighthouse of hope: the hope of building a pain medicine that does not evade uncertainty but crosses through it with courage, so as to help the many patients in pain who are lost in the ocean of a practice that too often rests on weak foundations. To offer, then, a light of courage and hope amid the darkness of human pain and suffering. I can think of no better reason for a clinician to undertake the journey that this book proposes.

University of A Coruña
A Coruña, Spain
ALFA FISIOTERAPIA, A Coruña, Spain
President of Galician Society of Physical Therapy (SOGAFI)
A Coruña, Spain
Eduardo Fondevila-Suárez, PT MSc
March 19, 2026

Preface

This Handbook has been written by two retired clinical and academic specialist pain medicine physicians, specifically to assist health professionals from diverse backgrounds to navigate many of the complex philosophical, theoretical, and practical issues that they will confront in the practice of this new but vital medical specialty. As we discovered over more than 30 years of *de facto* practice of pain medicine, before and since it became a specialty field in our native Australia, there is no readily accessible source of guidance about how one might think about these matters and therefore how one might translate any insights into practice.

These issues include philosophical dilemmas about the pain experience and the consequent difficulties with the language that is used on each side of the clinical encounter, and the different and not always complementary conceptual frameworks that are used for formulating and resolving clinical pain problems. There is a strong theme of epistemology, especially epistemic discipline, including insistence on accurate definition of constructs and identifying faulty reasoning. Particular attention is given to recurrent topics that are rarely discussed in the clinic, such as:

- The inherent uncertainty that attends the aporia of pain
- Conceptual frameworks versus explanatory models
- Intersubjectivity and the clinical encounter
- The salient role of nociception in the pain experience
- The challenge of rational clinical formulation

This Handbook is based on an edited compilation of material from our more than fifty peer-reviewed articles concerning theoretical and practical aspects of the specialty of Pain Medicine. It does not seek to be comprehensive, didactic, or prescriptive in a "how-to-do" sense, but rather to suggest "how-one-might-think-about" the issues. It contains ideas and syntheses that may be seen as new, challenging, or even controversial, with a view to being practical and accessible. The ultimate aim of this Handbook is improved quality of life for pain experiencers through enhanced effectiveness of their attending clinicians.

We gratefully acknowledge the major role played by various collaborators in our discussions and publications over a long time, including in particular Dr. David Buchanan (Australia), Dr. Simon van Rysewyk (Australia), and Dr. Asaf Weisman (Israel).

We would also acknowledge colleagues whose knowledge, experience, and wisdom have helped us formulate, hone, and develop the approaches that this Handbook presents, including in particular Dr. Geoffrey Bove (USA), Dr. David Champion (Australia), Melanie Galbraith (Australia), the late Dr. Brian Griffiths (Australia), Dr. Pamela Lyon (Australia), Emeritus Professor Horst Ruthrof (Australia), and Dr. Owen Williamson (Australia and Canada).

We are particularly grateful to Professor Eduardo Fondevila Suárez (Spain) for peer review of this manuscript and for contributing the Foreword.

Our thanks are also extended to Saki Kasai, Chihiro Haraguchi, Stephanie Sibin, and Ben Ingraham from *Springer Nature*, for expertly guiding us through the publication process.

Mosman, NSW, Australia
Mount Claremont, WA, Australia
February 2026

Milton L. Cohen
John L. Quintner

Contents

Trying to Gain Traction on a Slippery Subject 1

Clarifying the Definition of Pain 17

Chronic Pain: A Study in Language and Meaning 33

The Non-Convergent Language Used in Clinical and Taxonomic Settings . . . 45

Conceptual Frameworks 53

The Clinical (Two-Person) Encounter 69

The Salient Role of Nociception 89

Errors in Language and Logic Call for Epistemic Discipline 109

Case Studies in Tautology, Circular Reasoning and Conflation: Fibromyalgia and Myofascial Pain "Syndromes" 129

Translation into the Clinic 143

Appendix: Joint Peer-Reviewed Publications by the Authors 165

Trying to Gain Traction on a Slippery Subject

Abstract This chapter attempts to unbraid the complex twine that is "pain", identifying different strands, or conceptual windows, of aporia, experience, sensation, perception, emotion and reification. The IASP definitions of pain take for granted lay (English) connotations of sensation and perception, which do not align with an academic approach to the subject. This is intrinsically difficult, as pain is an aporia, an experience that is difficult to capture in language. As these perspectives are dissected, conflation between them is revealed, inevitably influencing theories of pain.

Two mutually incompatible consequences of this are identified. Firstly is the assertion that pain is an experience that does not require sensory input from the body, as captured in "neuromatrix theory" which can be refuted. Secondly is the reification of pain, that is, considering pain to be a "thing" that in turn can be an agent responsible for inducing physiological change, which is found to be an untenable concept.

Entrenchment of "pain-as-a-thing" in the literature has led to many misnomers, including "painful stimulus", "pain fibres" and "pain sensitivity", which are dissected and corrected, addressing another conflation of pain and nociception.

Some of the problems identified may be unresolvable, such as pain-as-an-aporia or the fundamental philosophical questions about pain which are formulated but not addressed here. However, other issues appear to be potentially resolvable, such as the problems of scientific language, especially concepts contingent upon pain-as-a-thing, distinguishing between pain, suffering and pain-related suffering, and anticipating the rebraiding of strands in the next chapter on definitively defining pain.

> It would be a great thing to understand Pain in all its meanings.
> Peter Mere Latham [1789–1875]. General Remarks on the Practice of Medicine, Ch XIV.

> Physical pain is not a simple affair of an impulse, travelling at a fixed rate along a nerve. It is the resultant of a conflict between a stimulus and the whole individual.
> Rene Leriche [1879–1955], Surgery of Pain, 1939.

Attempting to understand let alone define pain is daunting for a number of reasons. One is the conceptual challenge of making sense of the mystery of human experience that is pain; another is the linguistic challenge of how to express that experience accurately within the constraints of natural language (Cohen et al. 2018).

M. Cohen, J. Quintner, *A Philosophical Handbook for Pain Medicine Practice*,
https://doi.org/10.1007/978-981-92-1682-6_1

Other challenges arise from the different scientific conceptualisations of pain and the different approaches to its alleviation (Geniusas 2016:148):

- The physiologist seeks the underlying physical mechanisms of the observed phenomena (also called the "objective" side).
- The psychologist sees pain as a set of cognitive and emotive phenonema (also called the "subjective" side).
- Contemporary neuroscientists view pain as a neuro-chemical phenomenon.
- Anthropologists view pain through a socio-historical lens.
- Phenomenologists put these aside and focus instead on "how pain manifests itself not in someone else's, but in one's own personal experience".

Meanwhile, philosophers use the pain experience to explore various theories of philosophy of mind. This field is characterised by tension between the perspective of science and that of human experience, when it comes to how the mind and the world may be related.

This has been captured as the "Cartesian anxiety" (Bernstein 1983). On the one hand, there is a view, labelled "objectivist", that holds that "… there are or must be some fixed, permanent constraints to which we can appeal and which are secure and stable". On the other hand, the view, labelled "relativist", holds that "… there are no such basic constraints except those that we invent or temporally (and temporarily) accept" (Bernstein 1983). Then, "by treating the mind and the world as opposed subjective and objective poles, the Cartesian anxiety oscillates between the two in search of a ground" (Varela et al. 1993:141).

Tempting though it may be, it is beyond the scope of this Handbook to explore philosophy of mind any further.

However, when it comes to pain, perhaps the prime *philosophical* issues are expressed best in two questions as posed by Hardcastle (2017):

- "How is it that pain is both a sort of experience, but also the object of our experience?"
- "What sort of thing is pain such that it is private, subjective, and infallible, on the one hand, yet refers to things in the world about which we can be mistaken, on the other?" (p. 20)

This chapter does not seek to discuss let alone solve the complex problems inherent in these questions. Rather, it seeks to expand upon five perspectives of pain that confound the clinical encounter. These are:

- Pain as an aporia
- Pain as an experience
- Pain as a sensation

- Pain as an emotion
- Pain as a "thing"

Pain as an *Aporia*

To discuss "pain" is immediately to encounter an *aporia*. From the Greek meaning, "lacking a passage, a path, or a way", an aporia is "an expression of doubt, emerging when competing and compelling arguments are presented from both sides of a problem" (Murray 2009:9). Aporia encompasses the dual problems of not knowing how one has arrived here and not knowing where to go next (Burbules 2000).

Pain may be seen as an aporia, a mystery that defies us access to its secrets and complexities yet will not let us go away. Just when one feels that a concept of pain has been grasped, it slips away (Derrida 1994; Williamson et al. 2005). Nevertheless, it is necessary for clinicians to engage this aporia because of their ethical obligation to the person (as "the other") experiencing pain (Quintner et al. 2008).

The person in pain, also currently encountering the aporia, presents their body to the clinician for investigation and treatment with the quite reasonable expectation that the clinician will be able to "ground" their lived experience in scientific knowledge. But the clinician may also be denied access, so that both parties lack knowledge and understanding, which leads to crises of choice, of action and of identity.

Both patients and clinicians are trapped by the limitations of our language. We have tended to treat the pain of another person as if it existed as an independent reality ("a thing"). This practice serves only to generate explanations that are based upon our attempts to make sense and not upon those of the person experiencing pain. The inability to articulate and respond directly to the pain experience, however, introduces uncertainty into such explanations.

There is a divergence in the nature of the language that is used by pain experiencers and pain observers. The language use by the experiencer is likely to be in the domain of ontology, that is, there *exists* a phenomenon called pain, while that of the observer is in the domain of epistemology, that is, how can we *know* about that phenomenon (Williamson et al. 2005).

Although sensory and affective experiences are abstract concepts, "in the absence of real understanding or knowledge, the physiology of pain receives exquisite refinement instead. We talk about pain in the language of science, but the language of science remains, at bottom, the language of metaphor and 'as if' formulations masquerading as authoritative knowledge" (Neilson 2016:3).

Because a third-person observer cannot appreciate the first-person experience of another individual, the McGill Pain Questionnaire was developed in an attempt to bridge this gap (Melzack 1975; Melzack and Torgerson 1971). This questionnaire used the language of metaphor and "as if" formulations to reflect the many and varied sensory and emotional dimensions of pain.

The recognition that pain is an aporia and is beyond language should not engender a sense of clinical nihilism, but rather be a reminder that the use of language to denote and analyse the pain experience is imprecise and uncertain. All language-based paradigms are by their nature flawed to a greater or lesser extent.

When a somatic cause for pain is evident, the expected outcome is a reasonable degree of concordance between the observer's interpretations and those of the experiencer. However, when such a cause for pain cannot be located, both parties experience the failure of language to cope with the situation. Absence of "evidence" of pain is not evidence of absence of pain.[1]

These various problems and challenges cannot be solved here. What can—and indeed must—be addressed in a clinical handbook are not only the concepts employed by experiencers, observers and investigators of pain-related phenomena but also the words used to communicate them. The obvious starting point is the definition of pain.[2]

The International Association for the Study of Pain (IASP) has proposed two pragmatic definitions for the guidance of clinicians and researchers:

- 1979: An unpleasant sensory and emotional experience associated with actual or potential tissue damage or described in terms of such damage (IASP 1979).
- 2020: An unpleasant sensory and emotional experience associated with, or resembling that associated with, actual or potential tissue damage (Raja et al. 2020).

Both definitions presume familiarity of the pain community with the three key embedded concepts: experience, sensation and emotion. However, because the meanings of words are inherently fuzzy and changing, it needs to be acknowledged that these IASP definitions are lacking in clarity (Stoltz and Wood 2025).

Pain as an Experience

> All of our experiences of our life-world begin with bodily sensations which occur at the intersection of the person and their life-world. (Jarvis 2009:25)

Over time, the word "experience" has acquired an impressive range of meanings. Lexical definitions include:

- practical contact with and observation of facts or events
- particular instance of personally encountering or undergoing something
- the process or fact of personally observing, encountering or undergoing something
- the observing, encountering or undergoing of things generally as they occur in the course of time

[1] The "two-person" encounter will be discussed further in chapter, "The Clinical (Two-Person) Encounter".

[2] The definition of pain will be dissected in detail in chapter, "Clarifying the Definition of Pain". It is mentioned here to introduce the concepts of experience, sensation and emotion.

In broad terms, an experience can be defined as a personal encounter of, or with, something in the world (Paulsen 2020:863). It does need to be emphasised here that we have no voluntary control over our experiences (Bakhtin 1993:1). A pain experience is no exception; it simply "happens". However, for practical reasons, as will be developed in this Handbook, it may be most useful to consider the pain experience as a personal encounter with nociception.[3]

Is Pain a Sensation or a Perception?

Pain as a Sensation

A note to the first iteration of the IASP definition holds that pain is "unquestionably a sensation in a part or parts of the body" (IASP 1979). The revised definition does not contradict this assertion (Raja et al. 2020).

There is general agreement amongst scientists that sensations are primitive mental states induced by stimuli that may be external or internal to the body (Mather 2016:3).

The American Psychological Association (APA) defines sensation as an elementary state of consciousness that arises immediately after and as a result of the stimulation of a sense organ.[4] In this view, a sensation is a primal experience arising out of the activation of a specific apparatus and is not under conscious control. The sole function of sensations is to provide information to the organism.

Sensations have been divided into seven distinct modalities: audition, gustation, olfaction, somatosensation, balance, vision and nociception.[5] They differ in terms of the physical stimuli that excite their respective receptors, the neural structures involved in transduction and sensory analysis, and the specific information they convey. Importantly, the qualitative different modalities of sensation are "simply given" and are "essentially indescribable" (Lyon 2006). This is because they are subjective and due to the limitations of language imposed by pain (Scarry 1985:54).

---

[3] See chapter, "The Salient Role of Nociception".

[4] American Psychological Association Dictionary of Psychology—Perception. https://dictionary.apa.org/perception. Accessed 25.09.2023.

[5] In this list, nociception is a categorical outlier. "Audition" is the experience of hearing in response to a phonic stimulus; "gustation" and "olfaction" are respectively the experiences of tasting and smelling in response to a chemical stimulus; "somatosensation" is the experience of touch, pressure or movement in response to a physical stimulus; "vision" is the experience of seeing in response to a photic stimulus. By contrast, "nociception" does not describe an experience per se but rather is the organism's response to a noxious (= "tissue-damaging") stimulus. This is discussed in chapter, "Clarifying the Definition of Pain".

Pain as a Perception

By contrast, perception is the interpretation of information from the environment pertinent to identifying the meaning of the sensation. Sensation usually involves becoming aware of the existence of a stimulus, whereas perception involves the evaluation of the nature of the stimulus.[6]

Perception can have a dual meaning, being considered either as an intellectual operation that is purely mental in nature or as an operation mediated by the senses and involving the body. The genesis of confusion here is obvious.

Sensation or Perception?

As first pointed out by Boring (1933:6), to the experiencer, there is no introspective difference between a sensation and a perception (Millar 2017). Both take sensory stimulation as their starting point (Humphrey 2000).

While sensation then proceeds to represent the stimulation more or less as given, perception has to combine the evidence of stimulation with contextual information, memory and rules so as to construct a hypothetical model of the external world as it exists independently of the observer (Humphrey 2000).

As Humphrey specifies:

> We talk of "feeling" or "having" sensations - as if somehow sensations were the objects of our sensing, sense data, out there waiting for us to grasp them or observe them with our mind's eye. But analysis shows that this is a mistake. Sensations are no more the objects of sensing than, say, volitions are the objects of willing or intentions the objects of intending. (Humphrey 2000:8)

Therefore, the real importance of sensation is that it "lends a here-ness and a now-ness and a me-ness to the experience of the world, of which *pure perception in the absence of sensation is bereft*" (Emphasis added here) (Humphrey 1992:73). Rather than sensing being a passive state it is a form of active engagement with the stimulus occurring at the body surface:

> When, for example, I feel pain in my toe, or taste salt on my tongue, or equally when I have red sensation at my eye, I am in effect reaching out to the site of stimulation with a kind of evaluative response — a response appropriate to the stimulus and the body part affected. Indeed, what I experience as my sensation of "what is happening to me" is based not on the incoming information as such but rather on the signals I myself am issuing to make the response happen. This is how I feel about what's happening right now at my toe — I'm feeling painily about it. This is how I feel about what's happening right now at this part of the field of my eye — I'm feeling redly about it". (Humphrey 1992:9)

[6]American Psychological Association Dictionary of Psychology—Perception. https://dictionary.apa.org/perception. Accessed 25.09.2023.

It is important to note that neither the original nor the revised IASP definition of pain identifies a "perceptual" component, as each anchors that experience in the sensory and emotional dimensions only. Yet some pain theorists have conceptualised pain as a "pure" perception, begging the question of whether such an experience might be possible (Livingston 1953; Melzack 1961, 2001).

Such theorists have continued to use the term "perception", at times employing their own definitions but at other times not attempting to define it (Apkarian et al. 2005, 2013; Carlino and Benedetti 2016; Tabor et al. 2017). This recurring ambiguity in the pain literature poses a challenge to accuracy and consistency in usage (Goldberg et al. 2022).

Consider these usages:

- "Pain is a perception", which is solely an exercise in noun substitution without either being defined.
- "Pain perception" implies possible physiological processes involved in the perceptual domain, which remain unknown.
- "Perception of pain" implies that pain is "a thing". But pain is an experience and not a concrete objective entity that can be perceived (Cohen et al. 2022).

Regardless of any ambiguity in the existing definitions of perception, a consistent theme across all of them is the emphasis on perception as a cognitive construct that not only is quite distinct from peripheral sensory input but also does not necessarily require it. Therefore, it is all the more surprising that sensation and perception in the context of pain have become conflated.

Conflation[7] of Sensation and Perception

Conflation is the "collapsing of distinct items in such a way that their differences are apparently lost" (Haught 1995:13). The conflation fallacy occurs when they are treated as if they were the same, leading to confusion and potentially flawed reasoning. Haught refers to such an outcome of conflation as "an undifferentiated smudge" (p. 13).

The conflation of sensation and perception in psychology and neuroscience is particularly evident in the pain medicine literature, where one frequently encounters "a conceptual conflation between the process of sensation (where the world is sampled) and perception (whereby sensations are integrated with previous history and meaning)" (Pincus et al. 2007:626–7). This, as well as conflation with pain-as-emotion, can be traced to William Livingston (1953), a pioneering pain investigator who stated, "Pain, like all perceptions is subjective, individual and modified by degrees of attention, emotional states and the conditioning influence of past experiences".

[7] Conflation is a major theme in this Handbook.

Neuromatrix Theory

Canadian psychologist Ronald Melzack (1961), a leading figure in the pain world who had worked with Livingston, insisted that pain referred to a category of complex experiences but not to a specific sensation produced by a specific stimulus.

Using phantom limb phenomena as the example, Melzack (1990, 90) claimed that "neural networks within the brain generate all the qualities of experience that are felt to originate in the body; inputs from the body may trigger or modulate the output of the networks *but are not essential for any of the qualities of the experience*" (emphasis added here).

This was the essence of the body-self neuromatrix theory (Melzack 1990:91). Within this matrix, parts "are assumed to be specialized to process information related to major sensory events (such as injury) and may be termed neuromodules, which impress subsignatures on the larger neurosignature". This theory of pain integrated cognitive-evaluative (or "cognitive"), sensory-discriminative (or "sensory") and motivational affective (or "emotional") components, as had originally been proposed by Melzack and Casey (1968). A critical component of neuromatrix theory was the recognition that pain is "the consequence of the output of the widely distributed brain neural networks rather than a direct response to sensory input following tissue injury, inflammation and other pathologies".

Neuromatrix theory also asserted, strangely, "The body-self neuromatrix, however, *requires no actual sensory input to produce experiences of the body*" (Gatchel et al. 2007:584) (emphasis added here).

However, the neuroscientific assumptions for phantom limb pain and other phenomena that were used to underpin the neuromatrix theory of pain have long since been refuted (Rasminsky 1983). Nonetheless, the belief that the brain can generate a pain experience in the absence of nociceptive input persists, as a relic of neuromatrix theory. Fortunately, such a theory is not necessary in order to assert that that pain-as-a-sensation is altered cognitively (that is, through perception) and affectively (that is, through emotion) to result in pain-as-an-experience. Furthermore, a sensation, as a "given", can only be modulated "up" or "down", while perception is inherently malleable in many ways.

Pain as an Emotion

What Is an Emotion?

First and foremost, an emotion can be seen as both a mode of engagement in the world and a complex awareness of one's tendencies to act in it (Solomon 2008:10). Having an emotion (as opposed to just a simple "feeling") is an experience that embodies thoughts, judgements and other cognitive elements. Virtually, all emotions get expressed (however minimally) in behaviour (Solomon 2008).

Emotions can therefore be seen from a biological viewpoint as mental and bodily states that potentiate behaviour appropriate to environmental challenges (de Waal 2011). Following James (1884), de Waal (2011) conceptualised emotions as "an unlearned response system". In a similar vein, Barrett (2006) described an emotion as an orchestrated response to a significant event across multiple systems at once: perceptual, cognitive, motivational, expressive, bodily and experiential.

Deonna and Teroni (2015) located emotions at the level of attitudes or modes. In their opinion, emotions qualify as evaluations because they are a specific type of attitudes. These authors had previously argued the case for an attitudinal theory of emotions (Deonna and Teroni 2017). Their theory accounts for the observations that "emotions are triggered by events of some significance or relevance to an organism, that they encompass a coordinated set of changes in brain and body, and that they appear adaptive in the sense that they are directed towards coping with whatever challenge was posed by the triggering event" (Adolphs 2010:R549).

When a particular event arouses its interest, an organism rapidly evaluates its significance and decides whether action is needed. These reflex-like processes have been explored under the heading of *valence*.

What Is Valence?

Valence is a central component of all affective states, including pains, pleasures, emotions, moods and feelings of desire or repulsion (Carruthers 2018). It refers to an organism's capacity to assign a value (advantage/good, harm/bad) to a particular stimulus or the summary of information about its surroundings relative to its own current state (Lyon et al. 2021). Valence has been described as the most basic and original kind of subjective experience, "an instantaneous general feeling of one's state" (Veit 2022:288).

Valence appears to be pivotal to the evaluation of sensory stimuli, including those that induce nociception. This being the case, valence would constitute the emotional dimension of the pain experience as it plays a fundamental role in motivating all kinds of intentional action (Vazard 2024). However, the nature of emotional valence and the question of from where emotions draw their valence remain unresolved.

Why Is Pain Unpleasant?

A tentative explanation of the unpleasantness of the pain experience is that an organism's sensory inputs must be distinguishable from one another so that they can be evaluated and prioritised according to its immediate needs. The needs of an organism do not all carry equal weight. If this were not the case, those needs that are urgent in terms of its survival would not be prioritised (Lyon 2006). "Pain is more intolerable than thirst, which is more intolerable than hunger. That is because body trauma is more immediately critical for survival than either fluid or energy requirements" (Goodson 2003:91). The unpleasantness of pain can be seen to demand the attention of the organism when it has sustained bodily damage and immediate action is required (Veit 2023).

Pain as a Homeostatic Emotion?

Based on neurophysiological evidence in primates, Craig (2003:306) viewed pain in humans as "a homeostatic emotion reflecting an adverse condition in the body that requires a behavioural response".

The basic homeostatic "feelings", or modalities, include temperature, itch, visceral distension, muscle ache, hunger, thirst, "air hunger" and sensual touch. Each inherently generates an emotion that drives behaviour towards homeostasis whenever that is threatened.

In this view, pain is also a "homeostatic emotion", having originated from a physiological condition in the body that automatic (subconscious) homeostatic systems alone cannot rectify, and it comprises a sensation and a behavioural drive with reflexive autonomic adjustments. This raises the issue of pain being conceptualised as a "thing".

Pain as a "Thing"

In this Handbook, pain is conceptualised as an experience that has sensory, cognitive and emotional dimensions. This raises the issue of whether pain is a concrete entity—a "thing"—that has agency, that is, action or intervention producing a particular effect. In this respect, is pain an "input" or an "output"? This observer-dependent question is complex, controversial and possibly unanswerable. However, pain can also be seen as a biological process that the organism is undergoing when confronted with a threat to its integrity.

In the literature, pain-as-a-thing is the dominant discourse. Terms such as painful stimulus, pain nerves or fibres, pain sensitivity, pain threshold and pain tolerance abound. At first glance, these terms, often also used in lay parlance, may seem unexceptional. However, they are misnomers—"wrong names"—as they share the error of presuming that pain is a "thing" that is able to exert agency over other things (Cohen et al. 2022).

The definition of pain mentions an experience associated with, or resembling that associated with, actual or potential tissue damage. The IASP terminology does not define "tissue damage" but does recognise "a stimulus that is damaging or threatens damage to normal tissues" and labels that as a "noxious stimulus". So, it is valid to state that pain may be associated with a noxious stimulus (applied to the body). Pain, as an experience, is clearly a response and not a "thing"—an inanimate, material object—to which an organism might respond. It follows that it is not the stimulus that is "painful"; to assert otherwise is to court the circular argument that pain is an experience in response to a painful stimulus.[8]

The belief that pain is a "thing" with agency that can be held responsible for inducing physiological change is an example of the fallacy of presumption known as reification. The term reification is derived from the Latin *res* ("thing") and *facere* ("to make"). Reification is also known as the fallacy of misplaced concreteness, "the accidental error of mistaking the abstract for the concrete" (Whitehead 1925:58). Even using the term "experience of pain" implies that pain is a thing that evokes an experience. Pain *is* the experience, which is why this Handbook refers only and always to the "pain experience".

Similarly, "pain receptors", "pain nerves", "pain fibres" and "pain pathways" are misnomers, as they imply that pain is a message—a thing—transmitted by neural mechanisms from an origin to the brain. Nerve fibres and pathways are indeed required to electrically encode and transmit information following the activation of *nociceptors* that might occur in response to a noxious stimulus. That information also is not "pain", which is a whole-organism experience. The only correct terms for this neural substrate are "nociceptive nerves," "nociceptive fibres" and "nociceptive pathways".

Another example of how pain-as-a-thing has become entrenched in the language of the field is "pain sensitivity". This term appears to make sense because its connotation is the ability to tolerate pain, as in, "it takes a lot of stimulation for me to acknowledge that I am hurting", often incorrectly asserted as, "I have a high threshold for pain," when clearly that "threshold" has been surpassed. However, "pain sensitivity" is shorthand for "sensitivity to pain", the basic premise of which is that pain is a stimulus—a thing.

The pain experience is a response; "being sensitive" is itself a response; an organism cannot be "sensitive" to its own response.

It is noted that "pain sensitivity", "pain hypersensitivity" and "pain insensitivity" are not defined in the IASP terminology. Pain is not a "thing" to which an organism might be sensitive or insensitive or hypersensitive.

It has been argued here that the notion of pain as a concrete causative agent is untenable. On the other hand, the pain experience when seen as a process may cause an organism to change its behaviour. That experience however is mediated by nociception, as discussed in chapter, "The Salient Role of Nociception".

[8] Even the IASP terminology is not immune to this error. In the entry on *allodynia*, it is stated "The original modality [of stimulus] is normally nonpainful, but the response is painful", and there is mention of "a strong painful pinch to a normal person". *Pain threshold* is defined as "The minimum intensity of a stimulus that is perceived as painful", thus referring to the "noxiousness" of the stimulus whereas it is the person's *response* to the stimulus that defines their ability to tolerate it. This is discussed further in chapter, "Errors in Language and Logic Call for Epistemic Discipline", and chapter, "Translation into the Clinic".

Pain Versus Suffering

One way of conceptualising the pain experience is to dichotomise it into distress and disability. Each of these may be not only subjects of complaint from the pain experiencer but also objectively appreciated by a pain observer.[9] The distress component may arise from the sensory unpleasantness of the experience, the restrictions imposed on usual activity, and from the meaning or interpretation of the experiencer. This is often referred to as "suffering", captured succinctly by Cassell as "the state of severe distress associated with events that threaten the intactness of the person" (Cassell 1982).

However, "pain" and "suffering" tend to have been conflated. This situation has been abetted by the two iterations of the IASP definition of pain (above) which refer to the experience being "described in terms of such damage" (1979 iteration) or "resembling that associated with … damage" (2020 iteration). Two situations have arisen out of this. The first is the metaphorical use of pain to denote suffering, for example, the "pain" of having a "broken heart"; the second is that not all pain experiences are necessarily associated with suffering and not all suffering in a pain experiencer may be attributable to "damage".

There are at least two recent approaches to parsing these dilemmas. One is to reconceptualise the definitional association of pain away from "tissue damage" to the signalling to the organism that tissue damage has occurred or may occur, namely the process of nociception (Cohen et al. 2023; Weisman et al. 2026).[10] In this formulation "pain" refers only to that part of the experience that is attributable to nociception—perhaps a "bottom-up" view. The other approach—perhaps a "top-down" view—is the work that has been done to define pain-related suffering as "a severely negative, complex, and dynamic experience in response to a perceived threat to an individual's integrity as a self and identity as a person" (Noe-Steinmüller et al. 2024), conceptualised as related to but separate and distinct from pain (Stilwell et al. 2022).

To quote Coninx (2024):

> Chronic pain and suffering are two separate, albeit related experiences. Suffering, rather than pain, might be the driving factor for the distress and disability affecting many people in chronic pain … Furthermore, suffering is not solely determined by the persistence, sensory intensity, or unpleasantness of (chronic) pain. (p. 8)

This issue, of pain versus suffering, is discussed further in chapter, "Clarifying the Definition of Pain".

---

[9] This relationship will be dissected in chapter, "The Clinical (Two-Person) Encounter".

[10] See chapter, "The Salient Role of Nociception".

References

Adolphs R. Emotion. Curr Biol. 2010;20(3):R549–52. https://doi.org/10.1016/j.cub.2010.05.046.

Apkarian AV, Bushnell MC, Treede R-D, Zubieta J-K. Human brain mechanisms of pain perception and regulation in health and disease. Eur J Pain. 2005;9(4):463–84. https://doi.org/10.1016/j.ejpain.2004.11.001.

Apkarian AV, Baliki MN, Farmer MA. Predicting transition to chronic pain. Curr Opin Neurol. 2013;26(4):360–7. https://doi.org/10.1097/WCO.0b013e32836336ad.

Bakhtin MM. In: Liapunov V, Holquist M, editors. Toward a philosophy of the act (Vadim Liapunov, transl). Austin: University of Texas Press; 1993.

Barrett LF. Are emotions natural kinds? Perspect Psychol Sci. 2006;1:28–58. https://doi.org/10.1111/j.1745-6916.2006.00003.x.

Bernstein RJ. Beyond objectivism and relativism: science, hermeneutics and praxis. Philadelphia: University of Pennsylvania Press; 1983. p. 18.

Boring EG. The physical dimensions of consciousness. New York: The Century Co.; 1933.

Burbules NC. Aporias, webs and passages: doubt as an opportunity to learn. Curric Inq. 2000;30:171–87.

Carlino E, Benedetti F. Different contexts, different pains, different experiences. Neuroscience. 2016;338:19–26. https://doi.org/10.1016/j.neuroscience.2016.01.053.

Carruthers P. Valence and value. Philos Phenomenol Res. 2018;97:658–80. https://doi.org/10.1111/phpr.12395.

Cassell EJ. The nature of suffering and the goals of medicine. N Engl J Med. 1982;306:639–45.

Cohen M, Quintner J, van Rysewyk S. Reconsidering the international association for the study of pain definition of pain. Pain Rep. 2018;3(2):e634. https://doi.org/10.1097/PR9.0000000000000634.

Cohen ML, Weisman A, Quintner JL. Pain is not a "thing": how that error affects language and logic in pain medicine. J Pain. 2022;23(8):1283–93. https://doi.org/10.1016/j.jpain.2022.03.235.

Cohen ML, Quintner JL, Weisman A. "Nociplastic pain": a challenge to nosology and to nociception. J Pain. 2023;24(12):2131–9. https://doi.org/10.1016/j.pain.2023.07.019.

Coninx S. Pain philosophy: recent debates and future challenges. Philos Compass. 2024;19:e12981. https://doi.org/10.1111/phc3.12981.

Craig AD. A new view of pain as a homeostatic emotion. Trends Neurosci. 2003;26(6):303–7. https://doi.org/10.1016/S0166-2236(03)00123-1.

De Waal FBM. What is an animal emotion? Ann N Y Acad Sci. 2011;1224:191–206. https://doi.org/10.1111/j.1749-6632.2010.05912.4.

Deonna JA, Teroni F. Emotions as attitudes. Dialectica. 2015;69(3):293–311. https://doi.org/10.1111/1746-8361.12116.

Deonna JA, Teroni F. Getting bodily feelings into emotional experience in the right way. Emot Rev. 2017;9(1):55–63. https://doi.org/10.1177/175407391663966.

Derrida J. Aporias. Translated by Thomas Dutoit. Stanford: Stanford University Press; 1994.

Gatchel RJ, Peng YB, Peters ML, Fuchs PN, Turk DC. The biopsychosocial approach to chronic pain: scientific advances and future directions. Psychol Bull. 2007;133(4):581–624. https://doi.org/10.1037/0033-2909.133.4.581.

Geniusas S. Phenomenology of chronic pain: de-personalization and re-personalization. In: van Rysewyck S, editor. Meanings of pain. Cham: Springer International Publishing AG; 2016. p. 147–64. https://doi.org/10.1007/978-3-319-49022-9_9.

Goldberg B, Reuter K, Sytsma J. The history of the concept of pain: how the experts came to be out of touch with the folk. In: Hens K, De Block A, editors. Advances in experimental philosophy of medicine. Camden: Bloomsbury Publishing; 2022. p. 1–16.

Goodson FE. The evolution and function of cognition. Mahwah: Lawrence Erlbaum Associates, Inc.; 2003.

Hardcastle VG. A brief and potted overview on the philosophical theories of pain. In: Corns J, editor. The Routledge handbook of philosophy of pain. New York: Routledge; 2017. p. 19–28.

Haught JF. Science and religion: from conflict to conversation. New York: Paulist Press; 1995.
Humphrey N. A history of the mind: evolution and the birth of consciousness. New York: Simon and Schuster; 1992.
Humphrey N. The privatization of sensation. In: Huber L, Heyes C, editors. The evolution of cognition. Cambridge, MA: MIT Press; 2000. p. 241–52.
IASP. Pain terms: a list with definitions and notes on usage. Recommended by the IASP Subcommittee on taxonomy. Pain. 1979;6:247–52.
James W. What is an emotion? Mind. 1884;9:188–205.
Jarvis P. Learning to be a person in society: learning to be me. In: Illeris K, editor. Contemporary theories of learning. London: Routledge; 2009. p. 21–33.
Livingston WK. What is pain? Sci Am. 1953;188(3):59–67.
Lyon P. The biogenic approach to cognition. Cogn Process. 2006;7:11–29. https://doi.org/10.1007/s10339-005-0016-8.
Lyon P, Keijzer F, Arendt D, Levin M. Reframing cognition: getting down to biological basics. Philos Trans R Soc B. 2021;376:20190750. https://doi.org/10.1098/rstb.2019.0750.
Mather G. Foundations of sensation and perception. London: Psychology Press; 2016.
Melzack R. The perception of pain. Sci Am. 1961;204(2):41–9.
Melzack R. The McGill pain questionnaire: major properties and scoring methods. Pain. 1975;1:277–99. https://doi.org/10.1016/0304-3959(75)90044-5.
Melzack R. Phantom limbs and the concept of a neuromatrix. Trends Neurosci 1990;13(3):88-92. https://doi.org/10.1016/0166-2236(90)90179-E.
Melzack R. Pain and the neuromatrix in the brain. J Dent Educ. 2001;65:1378–82.
Melzack R, Casey KL. Sensory, motivational, and central control determinants of pain: a new conceptual model. In: Kenshalo D, editor. International symposium on the skin senses. Springfield: CC Thomas; 1968. p. 423–35.
Melzack R, Torgerson WS. On the language of pain. Anesthesiology. 1971;34:50–9. https://doi.org/10.1097/00000542-197101000-00017.
Millar B. Thinking with sensations. J Philos. 2017;114(3):134–54. https://doi.org/10.5840/jphil2017114311.
Murray SJ. Aporia: towards an ethic of critique. Aporia. 2009;1(1):8–14.
Neilson S. Pain as metaphor: metaphor and medicine. Med Humanit. 2016;42:3–10. https://doi.org/10.1136/medhum-2015-010672.
Noe-Steinmüller N, Scherbakov D, Zhuravlyov A, et al. Defining suffering in pain: a systematic review on pain-related suffering using natural language processing. Pain. 2024;2024(165):1434–49. https://doi.org/10.1097/j.pain.0000000000003195.
Paulsen MK. Appearance of experience as form and process. Integr Psych Behav. 2020;54:861–79. https://doi.org/10.1007/s12124-020-09526-3.
Pincus D, Freeman W, Modell A. A neurobiological model of perception: considerations for transference. Psychoanal Psychol. 2007;24(4):623–40. https://doi.org/10.1037/0736-9735.24.4.623.
Quintner JL, Buchanan D, Cohen ML, Katz J, Williamson O. Pain medicine and its models: helping or hindering? Pain Med. 2008;9:824–34. https://doi.org/10.1111/j.1526-4637.2007.00391.x.
Raja SN, Carr DB, Cohen M, Finnerup NB, Flor H, Gibson S, Keefe F, Mogil JS, Ringkam M, Sluka KA, Stevens B, Sullivan M, Tutelman P, Ushida T, Vader T. The revised IASP definition of pain: concepts, challenges, and compromise. Pain. 2020;161(9):1976–82. https://doi.org/10.1097/j.pain.0000000000001939.
Rasminsky M. Ectopic impulse generagtion in pathological nerve fibres. Trends Neurosci. 1983;6:388–90. https://doi.org/10.1016/0166-2236(83)90172-8.
Scarry E. The body in pain: the making and unmaking of the world. Oxford: Oxford University Press; 1985.
Solomon RC. The philosophy of emotions. In: Lewis M, Haviland-Jones JM, Barrett LF, editors. Handbook of emotions. 3rd ed. New York: The Guilford Press; 2008. p. 3–16.

Stilwell P, Hudon A, Meldrum K, et al. What is pain-related suffering? Conceptual critiques, key attributes, and outstanding questions. J Pain. 2022;23:729–38. https://doi.org/10.1016/j.jpain.2021.11.005.

Stoltz DS, Wood ML. Drawing out definitions. Am Sociol. 2025;56:396–416. https://doi.org/10.1007/s12108-024-09633-3.

Tabor A, Thacker MA, Moseley GL, Körding KP. Pain: a statistical account. PLoS Comput Biol. 2017;13(1):e1005142. https://doi.org/10.1371/journal.pcbi.1005142.

Varela FJ, Thompson E, Rosch E. The embodied mind. Cambridge, MA: The MIT Press; 1993. p. 140–3.

Vazard J. Feeling the unknown: emotions of uncertainty and their valence. Erkenntnis. 2024;89:1275–94. https://doi.org/10.1007/s10670-022-00583-1.

Veit W. The origins of consciousness or the war of the five dimensions. Biol Theor. 2022;17:276–91. https://doi.org/10.1007/s13752-022-00408-y.

Veit W. Complexity and the evolution of consciousness. Biol Theor. 2023;18:175–90. https://doi.org/10.1007/s13752-022-00407-z.

Weisman A, Quintner J, Cohen M. Adieu to an aphorism: why nociception is necessary for pain. Brain. 2026;149(2):422–31. https://doi.org/10.1093/brain/awaf387.

Whitehead AN. Science and the modern world. New York: MacMillan Company; 1925.

Williamson OD, Buchanan DA, Quintner JL, Cohen ML. Pain beyond monism and dualism. Pain. 2005;116(1):169–70. https://doi.org/10.1016/j.pain.2005.04.011.

Clarifying the Definition of Pain

Abstract The evolution of the definitions of pain developed by the International Association for the Study of Pain (IASP) is presented and analysed. This evolution culminated in the 2020 iteration: "Pain is an unpleasant sensory and emotional experience associated with, or resembling that associated with, actual or potential tissue damage".

However, a compound paradox has been identified in this revised definition of pain, such that it simultaneously prescribes a connection between pain and tissue damage and allows that prescription to be violated. The first paradox is that contradictory true positions can be held, when the experiencer claims to be "in pain" and the observer cannot find the required association with tissue damage or, preferably as is argued, nociception. The second paradox is revealed by the construct of "nociplastic" pain, which contradicts the IASP definition to the extent that nociceptors have not been activated, yet at the same time is consistent with that definition to the extent that it "resembles" an experience associated with actual or potential tissue damage.

The IASP definition of pain can be strengthened by removing the current ambiguity of interpretation, grounding the experience in a reconceptualisation of nociception as activation of a nociceptive apparatus, and clearly distinguishing it from suffering. The offered clarifying definition is: Pain is a mutually recognised experience contingent upon nociception.

Defining "Pain"

The modern formulation of a definition of pain began with Merskey (1964):

> An unpleasant experience which we primarily associate with tissue damage or describe in terms of such damage, or both.

This definition conceptualised pain as (a) an experience that is (b) associated with tissue damage.

A number of other versions followed, based on the same structure (Table 1).

M. Cohen, J. Quintner, *A Philosophical Handbook for Pain Medicine Practice*, https://doi.org/10.1007/978-981-92-1682-6_2

Table 1 Versions of a definition of pain, 1968–2020

Formulation	Comment
Sternbach (1968): "Pain" denotes (i) a personal, private sensation of hurt, (ii) a harmful stimulus which signals current or impending tissue damage, and (iii) a pattern of responses which operate to protect the organism from harm	Conflates a stimulus ("harmful"), a sensation ("hurt") and a teleological function ("to protect the organism")
Melzack (1973): "Pain" represents "a category of experiences, signifying a multitude of different unique events having different causes, and characterised by different qualities along a number of sensory and affective dimensions"	Tautological
Mountcastle (1974): Pain is "that sensory experience evoked by stimuli that injure or threaten to destroy tissue, defined introspectively by every [man] as that which hurts"	Circular argument: "pain is that which hurts" Experience tied to an alarming stimulus ("threaten to destroy")
Fabrega and Tyma (1976): Pain is an unpleasant perception which the individual explicitly refers to [his] body and which can represent a form of suffering	Pain as a perception Somatic location Separate from suffering
IASP (1979): "An unpleasant sensory and emotional experience associated with actual or potential tissue damage, or described in terms of such damage"	See text
Olivier (2008): Pain is disturbed bodily perception bound to hurt, affliction, or agony	Mode of bodily perception "Hurt", "agony" and "affliction" require definition Does "bound to" mean "tied to" or "destined to"?
Wright (2011): Pain is the (sic) unpleasant sensation that has evolved to motivate behaviour, which avoids or minimises tissue damage, or promotes recovery	Presumed evolutionary role Implicit association with tissue damage
Smith et al. (2011) An unpleasant experience on the part of a human subject that is both sensory and emotional and is of a type that is either canonical pain or phenomenologically indistinguishable from canonical pain [Note added in article: "canonical" pain occurs in response to, and is concordant with, tissue damage and is, in evolutionary terms, the most basic case of pain from which all other pains were to be seen as variant phenomena]	It is unclear how pain that is "phenomenologically indistinguishable from canonical pain" is not in fact "canonical pain"
Price and Barrell (2012): The phenomenology of pain is based on (i) its unique sensory qualities; (ii) a meaning of intrusion or threat; and (iii) related feelings of unpleasantness or other negative emotions	Formulation resembles diagnostic criteria for a syndrome or a disease rather than being a definition

(continued)

Table 1 (Continued)

Formulation	Comment
Aydede (2016): An unpleasant sensory and emotional experience that results from actual or impending tissue damage, or is correctly describable in terms of such damage	Explicit association with tissue damage Who determines the "correctness" of a person's description of pain?
Williams and Craig (2016): Pain is a distressing experience associated with actual or potential tissue damage with sensory, emotional, cognitive and social components	Adding "cognitive" and "social" components to the definition does not clarify the relationship between "tissue damage" and the pain experience
Cohen et al. (2018): Pain is a mutually recognisable somatic experience that reflects a person's apprehension of threat to their bodily or existential integrity	Mutual recognition Privileges neither experiencer nor observer Moves from "damage" to "threat to integrity" Does not distinguish well enough between pain and related suffering
Raja et al. (2020): "An unpleasant sensory and emotional experience associated with, or resembling that associated with, actual or potential tissue damage"	Minimal change from 1979 definition: "described in terms of such damage" substituted with "resembling that associated with [damage]"

In order to identify the fundamental attributes of a definition of pain that might underlie these formulations, it is also useful to review the Note that accompanied the 1979 IASP iteration. The clauses of the Note are numbered here, in the order in which they appeared in a single paragraph at publication:

(i) The inability to communicate verbally does not negate the possibility that an individual is experiencing pain and is in need of appropriate pain-relieving treatment.
(ii) Pain is always subjective.
(iii) Each individual learns the application of the word through experiences related to injury in early life.
(iv) Biologists recognize that those stimuli which cause pain are liable to damage tissue.
(v) Accordingly, pain is that experience we associate with actual or potential tissue damage.
(vi) It is unquestionably a sensation in a part or parts of the body, but it is also always unpleasant and therefore also an emotional experience.
(vii) Experiences which resemble pain but are not unpleasant, e.g., pricking, should not be called pain.
(viii) Unpleasant abnormal experiences (dysesthesias) may also be pain but are not necessarily so because, subjectively, they may not have the usual sensory qualities of pain.
(ix) Many people report pain in the absence of tissue damage or any likely pathophysiological cause; usually this happens for psychological reasons.

(x) There is usually no way to distinguish their experience from that due to tissue damage if we take the subjective report.
(xi) If they regard their experience as pain, and if they report it in the same ways as pain caused by tissue damage, it should be accepted as pain.
(xii) This definition avoids tying pain to the stimulus.
(xiii) Activity induced in the nociceptor and nociceptive pathways by a noxious stimulus is not pain, which is always a psychological state, even though we may well appreciate that pain most often has a proximate physical cause.

Attributes that can be extracted here are:

Subjectivity (experiencer-dependency)	Clauses ii, vi, viii, x, xi
Association with tissue damage (note that clause xii in fact contradicts this)	Clauses iv, v, xi
Nociception is not pain	Clause xiii
Pain without tissue damage is "psychological"	Clause ix

In 2020, the IASP definition of pain was revised,

from an unpleasant sensory and emotional experience associated with actual or potential tissue damage, or described in terms of such damage

to an unpleasant sensory and emotional experience associated with, or resembling that associated with, actual or potential tissue damage [D].

Both these iterations:

- have perpetuated the association with tissue damage (even though "tissue damage" is not defined);
- have privileged the view of the experiencer over that of the observer: "described in terms of such damage" and "resembling that associated with … damage", although to the continuing disadvantage of non-verbal beings; and
- have ignored dissatisfaction with the adjective "unpleasant", which neither captures the experience for many people nor distinguishes pain from other unpleasant experiences.

However, the Notes[1] that accompany the 2020 iteration do help to clarify some potential ambiguities:

1. Pain is always a personal experience that is influenced to varying degrees by biological, psychological and social factors.
2. Pain and nociception are different phenomena. Pain cannot be inferred solely from activity in sensory neurons.

[1] Each note is given a number here, to facilitate future reference.

3. Through their life experiences, individuals learn the concept of pain.
4. A person's report of an experience as pain should be respected.
5. Although pain usually serves an adaptive role, it may have adverse effects on function and social and psychological well-being.
6. Verbal description is only one of several behaviours to express pain; inability to communicate does not negate the possibility that a human or a nonhuman animal experiences pain.

These Notes situate the revised definition more firmly in a biopsychosocial conceptual framework[2] and make the important distinction between pain and nociception, yet continue to equivocate about the interpretation of "a person's report of an experience as pain". This will be explored below.

Unexpected Paradoxes in the IASP Definition

In chapter "Trying to Gain Traction on a Slippery Subject", the "prime paradox" of pain was mentioned, well expressed in the two questions posed by Hardcastle (2017):

- "How is it that pain is both a sort of experience but also the object of our experience?"
- "What sort of thing is pain such that it is private, subjective, and infallible on the one hand, yet refers to things in the world about which we can be mistaken on the other?"

Furthermore, in English, the one and the same word is used for both the experience itself and the object of that experience. This has been succinctly expressed by Bradley (2021):

> The truth is that we use the expression "pain" (and related expressions such as "hurts") in many different ways. In English we say, for instance, that a body part *hurts* or *has a pain in it*, that a person is *in pain* or is *feeling pain*, or that a psychological state *is painful*. (Italics in original)

It does seem that, in the English language, too much is asked of one word—"pain"—to accommodate philosophical, biological, clinical and taxonomic perspectives.

Recently, it has been shown that the 2020 iteration of the IASP definition of pain contains a compound paradox, such that *it simultaneously prescribes a connection between pain and tissue damage and allows that prescription to be violated* (Cohen et al. 2026). The discussion to follow presents these paradoxes and indicates that this definition can be strengthened by removing the current ambiguity of interpretation, grounding the pain experience in a reconceptualisation of nociception, and clearly distinguishing it from suffering.

---

[2] See chapter "Conceptual Frameworks".

The Definitional Association of the Pain Experience with Tissue Damage

As shown above, both the 1979 and 2020 definitions prescribe a nexus—"associated with"—between pain and tissue damage. In effect, this grounds the subjective experience in the objective reality of tissue damage, which is not defined in the IASP lexicon. In effect, the only difference between these two definitions is the substitution of "resembling" for "described in terms of" with respect to the association with tissue damage.

However, each of these definitions in fact consists of four non-identical sub-definitions, arising out of the disjunctive conjunction "or" being used twice. To use the 2020 iteration, these are:

[D-i] Pain is an unpleasant sensory and emotional experience associated with actual tissue damage.

[D-ii] Pain is an unpleasant sensory and emotional experience associated with potential tissue damage.

[D-iii] Pain is an unpleasant sensory and emotional experience resembling that associated with actual tissue damage.

[D-iv] Pain is an unpleasant sensory and emotional experience resembling that associated with potential tissue damage.

The question then arises, is each one of these four experiences phenomenologically equivalent to each of the others? For example, do [D-i] and [D-iv] define the same experience, especially when seen from the viewpoint of scientific enquiry and therefore clinical application?

Sub-definition [D-i] is uncontroversial, as it reflects the common and common-sense-derived situation that a mutually recognisable experience that is labelled as "pain" often occurs when a body part has been damaged, whether that be due to trauma or disease.

Furthermore, in logical terms, sub-definition [D-i] is equivalent to stating that a reported pain experience implies that actual tissue damage has occurred.

The Paradox Posed by Discordant Views

This issue of assocation raises two important questions:

- Who determines whether there is an association with tissue damage?
- By whom and how is the "resembling" to that association to be determined?

Before discussing those questions, the issue of "actual" and "potential" tissue damage needs to be addressed.

"Actual" vs. "Potential"

Actual tissue damage (sub-definition [D-i]) poses no problem when it is obvious. However, what would be meant by "potential" tissue damage, that is, damage that might eventuate but has not yet occurred? Does that denote (a) a possible response to a stimulus that is currently not tissue-damaging but may become noxious, (b) a situation where tissue damage is imminent but has not yet occurred or (c) an apprehension that tissue damage might occur? These are three examples reflecting that "potential" in fact includes all possibilities and therefore specifies none of them, thus defying definition. The only relevant event then is *actual* tissue damage (which remains undefined).

It follows that the "actual or potential" qualification should be removed, so that a new formulation of definition [D] would refer only to "tissue damage", with only two sub-definitions:

[D-i] Pain is an unpleasant sensory and emotional experience associated with tissue damage.

[D-iii] Pain is an unpleasant sensory and emotional experience resembling that associated with tissue damage.

That leads to consideration of "resembling".

"Resembling"

> If they regard their experience as pain and if they report it in the same ways as pain caused by tissue damage, it should be accepted as pain.
> (Note xi to the 1979 IASP definition of pain, as above)

This Note, often rendered as "Pain is what the person says it is", appears to have circumscribed what is to be connoted by "pain", even more than the wording of the definition itself. The Note to the 2020 definition is a little less generous: "A person's report of an experience as pain should be respected" (Raja et al. 2020).

If "pain is what the person says it is", then how would it ever be possible to deny an assertion of pain? A nihilistic response would be, why would one even bother to attempt to define pain? Clearly, for scientific and clinical purposes, if not also for its moral, legal and philosophical implications, an attempt to define pain, despite the difficulties that attend an aporia,[3] is necessary and desirable.

This issue of determining "resembling" comes down to the contrast between an experiencer's view and an observer's view of the phenomenon.

Can an observer know what the other person is experiencing? In the ordinary sense of "knowing", observers can and commonly do appreciate that another person is experiencing pain through observing the other's language and/or behaviour and integrating that with their own experience and learning. This is the essence of the "mutually recognisable" qualifier proposed in the table above (Cohen et al. 2018).

---

[3] See chapter "Trying to Gain Traction on a Slippery Subject".

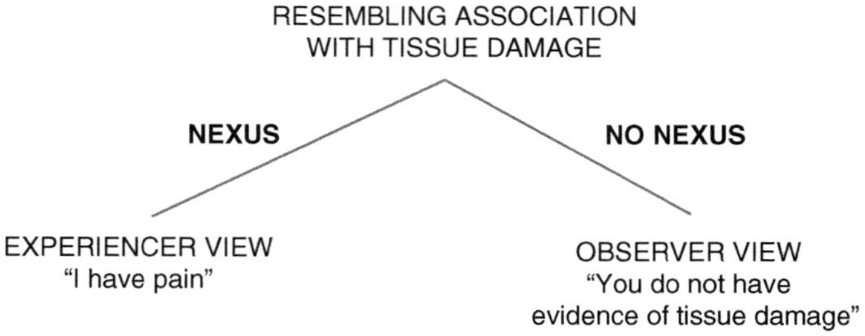

Fig. 1 First example of simultaneously valid contradictory views

However, an observer may never know with certainty whether the experiencer is making the definitional association between the pain experience and tissue damage. In situation [D-iii] above (pain is an unpleasant sensory and emotional experience resembling that associated with actual tissue damage), who determines the "resembling", the experiencer or the observer?

- The experiencer might say, "It feels as if there is a knife in my back", the implication being that tissue damage is occurring there.
- The observer might say, "On the basis of observing their language and behaviour, this person's distress is as if there were tissue damage occurring in their back".

But what if the observer—specifically a clinician—were to assert, "Despite it appearing that there is tissue damage occurring in this person's back, I can find no evidence thereof".

This is the first paradox. The experiencer maintains a belief that there must be tissue damage, while the observer can find no somatic corroboration for that assertion. Although contradictory, both views are simultaneously valid (Fig. 1).

Which view is to prevail? If it is that of the experiencer, as was one of the principles laid down for the 2020 revision, then there is neither a need nor a possibility for a definition, as any subjective assertion qualifies—"pain is anything that hurts" (Treede 2018).

Mention was made above of the Notes that accompany the 2020 definition, including "A person's report of an experience as pain should be respected" (Raja et al. 2020). However, "respecting" a report of a pain experience is not the same as accepting or believing it. This stipulation to respect a report is not violated at all by the argument being put forward, as the dialogue now becomes:

- Experiencer: "I (believe that I) have tissue damage (causing my pain)".
- Clinician-observer: "You do not have evidence of tissue damage, and therefore, your distress, which I respect, is not concordant with the accepted definition of 'pain.' We need to find another explanation for your distress".

It is argued that a truly scientific resolution of this paradox can be determined only by allowing the observer's view to prevail. That would privilege sub-proposition [D-i] over [D-iii].

The Paradox Posed by "Nociplastic Pain"

In 2016, the construct of "nociplastic" pain was developed, to account for patients whose pain could not attract either of the then current 2011 descriptors, "nociceptive" or "neuropathic".[4] Nonetheless, these patients demonstrate clinical and psychophysical hypersensitivity to non-noxious stimuli applied to apparently normal tissues in the region of their pain. The inescapable inference is that in these patients a change in nociceptive function has occurred.

Nociplastic pain has been formally defined as "Pain that arises from altered nociception despite no clear evidence of actual or threatened tissue damage causing the activation of peripheral nociceptors or evidence for disease or lesion of the somatosensory system causing the pain" (Kosek et al. 2016). In this definition, "nociception" specifically refers to the IASP formulation, "the neural process of encoding noxious stimuli". In other words, "nociplastic pain" occurs in the absence of nociception-as-currently-defined (NACD).

To the extent that nociplastic pain cannot be demonstrated to be associated with NACD, then "nociplastic pain" is "not-pain". However, at the same time, "nociplastic pain" does conform to the definition of pain, as in sub-definition [D-iii] to the degree that it "resembles" [D-i].

This is the second paradox in the IASP definition, that "nociplastic pain" is simultaneously consistent with, yet contradictory to, the definition of pain (Fig. 2).

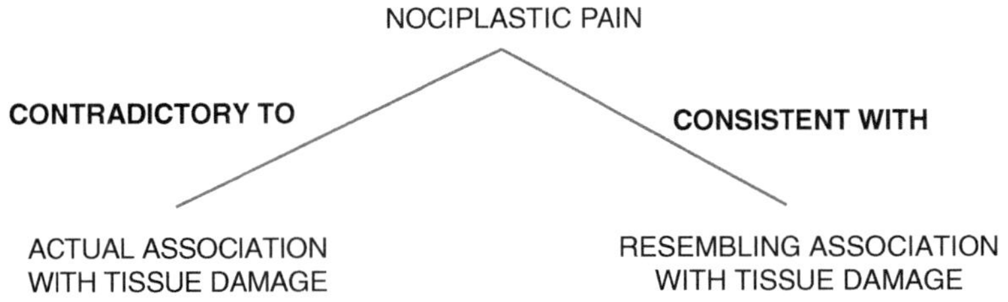

Fig. 2 Second example of simultaneously valid contradictory views

[4] These termed are discussed in chapter "The Salient Role of Nociception". It should be noted that "pain descriptor" is a misnomer, as the terms are hypotheses of nociception. This is a prime example of conflation between pain and nociception.

Resolution of this Situation

To reiterate, unintentionally embedded in the IASP definition of pain is the paradox that it simultaneously prescribes a connection between pain and tissue damage yet allows that connection to be violated. The contradiction that constitutes this paradox is the inability to resolve the issue where there is discordance between the pain experiencer and the observer, in which the former relies on "resembling" the definitional connection while the latter relies on finding evidence of tissue damage.

Resolving the Paradox of Discordant Views

It has been identified that the assertions, "Pain is what the person says it is" and "If they regard their experience as pain and if they report it in the same ways as pain caused by tissue damage, it should be accepted as pain", lead to an untenable paradox of interpretation of the definition of pain, when an experience "resembling" one associated with tissue damage (sub-definition [D-iii]) is given weight equal to one that is associated with tissue damage (sub-definition [D-i]).

The most straight-forward solution would be use use [D-i] as a definitive new version, namely,

[P] Pain is an unpleasant sensory and emotional experience associated with tissue damage, but with a new requirement that "tissue damage" be defined, which would also entail how that is to be determined, and therefore by whom.

This solution challenges a principle that has always been a basis for the IASP approach, namely that of privileging the view of the pain experiencer over that of the observer. To have a definition that, in effect, makes it impossible to say that a reported experience is not pain serves neither taxonomic nor operational purposes.

Proposition [P] is equivalent to stating that the complaint of pain implies that tissue damage has occurred. The onus of application then shifts onto the observer to determine that latter phenomenon. Put formally, that is to privilege the view of the clinical observer over that of the experiencer. As exemplified above, this stance in effect maintains respect for the experiencer's point of view while adhering to the definitional connection between pain and tissue damage.

This point raises the question of pain-related suffering as was discussed in chapter "Trying to Gain Traction on a Slippery Subject", and summarised in this quote from Coninx (2024):

> Chronic pain and suffering are two separate, albeit related experiences. Suffering, rather than pain, might be the driving factor for the distress and disability affecting many people in chronic pain … Furthermore, suffering is not solely determined by the persistence, sensory intensity, or unpleasantness of (chronic) pain. (p. 8)

In fact, the stance entailed in proposition [P] above may in effect enhance the clinician's appreciation of the other person's suffering. This further highlights the potential utility of making a clear distinction between the pain experience and suffering.

Resolving the Paradox Posed by Nociplastic Pain

The deliberations of the IASP Task Force that developed the revised 2020 definition ([D] above) made it clear that the link with tissue damage was not negotiable. However, proposition [P] does not deal with the challenge posed by the "nociplastic" construct.

"Nociplastic" is part of the IASP terminology that turns on the adjective "noxious", which generally means "harmful" or "injurious".[5] In the IASP lexicon, "noxious" is defined only in the context of a "noxious stimulus" as one "that is damaging or threatens damage to normal tissues" (IASP 1979). The Note to the 1979 iteration and the Notes that accompany the 2020 iteration do refer to *nociceptor* and *nociception*,[6] derived from the same root.

However, there is no noun in English corresponding to "noxious". In any event, it is not the event of tissue damage itself that is important to the organism but rather the signalling to the organism that a noxious event is occurring. Therefore, it is argued that it is valid to extrapolate from tissue damage to the signalling thereof, properly termed nociception, formally defined by the IASP as "the neural process of encoding noxious stimuli" (IASP 1979).

Proposition [P] could then be recast as:

[Q] Pain is an unpleasant sensory and emotional experience associated with nociception.

This maintains the connection in the definition by inserting a definable link—the signalling of tissue damage, namely "nociception"—between the undefined "tissue damage" and the pain experience. Thus, the *intent* of the definition is not compromised. Such a change in focus, from the externality of a noxious event to how the organism might respond to such an event, entails a more biologically based approach.

However, to accommodate the clinical phenomena that lead to the construct of "nociplastic pain", that approach requires a broader concept of nociception than the current "neural process of encoding noxious stimuli", which considers only peripheral activation of nociceptors, towards that of activation of a nociceptive apparatus,[7] reflecting the interaction of that neuronal substrate with cellular and

[5] From the Latin "nocere", to hurt; "noxa", injury, hurt or damage; "noxius", hurtful, injurious.

[6] These terms and others in the IASP lexicon will be discussed in chapter "The Salient Role of Nociception".

[7] "Nociceptive apparatus" will be discussed in chapter "The Salient Role of Nociception".

humoral elements of the immune system (Cohen et al. 2023). Both neuroanatomical (Coghill 2020) and physiological (Grimm 2025) bases for such an apparatus have been proposed.

The onus of application of proposition [Q] remains with the observer to determine the presence of activation of the nociceptive apparatus. As exemplified above, this approach maintains respect for the experiencer's point of view while adhering to the definitional connection between pain and nociception.

The Issue of Causation

The current definition [D] and propositions [P] and [Q] can still be seen to hedge the question of whether the "association" of pain with tissue damage/nociception is causal.

The Note accompanying the 1979 definition of pain included the following clause (as identified by Roman numerals above):
(xiii; first part)

"Activity induced in the nociceptor and nociceptive pathways by a noxious stimulus is not pain ..."

This has been stated more explicitly and simply in the second Note to the revised (2020) definition (as numbered in Arabic numerals above):

(2) "Pain and nociception are different phenomena: the experience of pain cannot be reduced to activity in sensory neurons" (Raja et al. 2020).

Put another way, this means that nociception may not lead to pain or, in causal language, nociception is not sufficient for pain.

The Note to the 1979 definition (IASP 1979) also stated (clauses as numbered above):

(ix) "Many people report pain in the absence of tissue damage or any likely pathophysiological cause; usually (*sic*) this happens for psychological (*sic*) reasons".
(xii) "This definition avoids tying pain to the stimulus".
(xiii; second part)

"... pain, which is always a psychological state, even though we may well appreciate that pain *most often has a proximate physical cause*". (Emphasis added here.)

Clauses (xii) and (xiii; second part) above are contradictory. Despite that, clauses (ix) and (xii) together have led to the assertion that pain may occur in the absence of nociception or, in causal language, nociception is not necessary for pain. However, that assertion clearly contradicts the current definition of pain.

If "... pain most often has as a proximate proximate physical cause" is taken as a definitive statement, then the "proximate physical cause" of pain that occurs "most often" can only be tissue damage or, preferably, nociception. Indeed the coincidence of nociception and pain is ubiquitous: not only is nociception associated with the majority of instances of pain but also nociception precedes pain, not the reverse. That is, a pain experience relies on the prior presence of nociception, even if pain does not always ensue. In causal language, *nociception is necessary for pain.*[8]

This inference, which can be made from the current definition of pain, has been supported in a recent review that has found no confident demonstration, clinically or experimentally, of pain experienced or induced in the absence of nociception (Weisman et al. 2026).

Proposed Modifications of the IASP Definition of Pain

The revised IASP definition of pain (Raja et al. 2020) has been shown to contain two paradoxes, which together reveal that it simultaneously prescribes a connection between pain and tissue damage and allows that prescription to be violated.

This situation is unacceptable in a definition that seeks to provide a basis for scientific enquiry and clinical practice. That definition never sought to resolve the philosophical paradox and does not, on its own, provide a taxonomical way of distinguishing "pain" from "non-pain". It has been shown here to have failed in an operational role, as on the one hand it allows pain to be "what the person says it is", while on the other hand it does not enforce its definitional nexus with a biologically based objective reality.

Therefore, for clinical and scientific purposes, and with no claim of utility for the philosophers' problem with pain as mentioned above, a first modification of the IASP definition is proposed to:

[Q] Pain is an unpleasant sensory and emotional experience associated with nociception, with the vital caveat that nociception itself needs to be redefined[9] (Cohen et al. 2026).

However, considering the causal argument made above, that nociception is necessary for pain, it is no longer appropriate to continue to use the phrase "associated with" in the definition. Therefore, a second modification of the definition can be proposed to:

[R] Pain is an unpleasant sensory and emotional experience contingent on nociception, with nociception being reconceptualised as above (Cohen et al. 2026).

[8] See extensive discussion in chapter "The Salient Role of Nociception".

[9] Reconceptualisation of nociception as "activation of a neuronal apparatus that is capable of responding to a noxious stimulus" is discussed in chapter "The Salient Role of Nociception".

Consistent with an earlier proposal (Cohen et al. 2018), this proposition could be modified further to:

[S] Pain is a mutually recognised experience contingent on nociception, with the caveat as above (Cohen et al. 2026).

These proposals, based on logical and biological argument, remove the current ambiguity of interpretation by grounding the pain experience in a reconceptualisation of nociception, thus making a clear distinction between that experience and nociception on the one hand and suffering on the other. This grounding not only enhances the observer's respect for the experiencer in the clinical encounter but also lays the foundation for distinct therapeutic approaches to those three elements.

Definitions do not only underpin clinical practice but also actively construct it, determining how pain is mutually understood, assessed and addressed in the consulting room. The clinical encounter itself depends on definitions, as every interaction involves fundamental assumptions about the relationship between subjective reports and objective findings, the legitimacy of personal experience, and the difficulty of dealing with the aporia of pain.[10]

References

Aydede M. Defending the IASP definition of pain. Monist. 2016;3(2):1–28. https://doi.org/10.1093/monist/onx021.

Bradley A. The paradox of pain. Philos Q. 2021;71:717–37. https://doi.org/10.1093/PQ/PQAA084.

Coghill RC. The distributed nociceptive system—a framework for understanding pain. Trends Neurosci. 2020;43(10):780–94. https://doi.org/10.1016/j.tins.2020.07.004.

Cohen M, Quintner J, van Rysewyck S. Reconsidering the IASP definition of pain. Pain Rep. 2018;3(2):e634. https://doi.org/10.1097/PR9.0000000000000634.

Cohen M, Quintner J, Weisman A. "Nociplastic pain": a challenge to nosology and to nociception. J Pain. 2023;24:2131–9. https://doi.org/10.1016/j.jpain.2023.07.019.

Cohen ML, Weisman A, Quintner JL. Paradoxes weaken the IASP definition of pain. Korean J Pain. 2026;39(1):1–8. https://doi.org/10.3344/kjp.25268.

Coninx S. Pain philosophy: recent debates and future challenges. Philos Compass. 2024;19:e12981. https://doi.org/10.1111/phc3.12981.

Fabrega J Jr, Tyma S. Language and cultural influences on the description of pain. J Psychosom Res. 1976;20:323–37. https://doi.org/10.1111/j.2044-8341.1976.tb02387.x.

Grimm HM. The role of the immune system in nociception development: a neuroimmune perspective. Sci Insights. 2025;46(4):1795–8. https://doi.org/10.15354/si.25.op269.

Hardcastle VG. A brief and potted overview on the philosophical theories of pain. In: Corns J, editor. The Routledge handbook of philosophy of pain. New York: Routledge; 2017. p. 19–28.

IASP. Pain terms: a list with definitions and notes on usage: recommended by the IASP Subcommittee on taxonomy. Pain. 1979;6:249.

Kosek E, Cohen M, Baron R, Gebhart GF, Mico J-A, Rice AS, Rief W, Sluka KA. Do we need a third mechanistic descriptor for chronic pain states? Pain. 2016;157:1382–6. https://doi.org/10.1097/j.pain.0000000000000507.

[10] See chapter "The Clinical (Two-Person) Encounter".

Melzack R. The puzzle of pain. New York: Basic Books; 1973.
Merskey H. An investigation of pain in psychological illness. D.M thesis. Oxford. 1964.
Mountcastle VB. Pain and temperature sensibilities. In: Mountcastle VB, editor. Medical physiology. 13th ed. Saint Louis: Mosby; 1974. p. 341–81.
Olivier A. The problem of defining pain. Philos Today. 2008;52:3–14. https://doi.org/10.5840/philtoday200852136.
Price DD, Barrell JJ. Inner experiences and neuroscience. Merging the two perspectives. Cambridge, MA: MIT Press; 2012.
Raja SN, Carr DB, Cohen M, Finnerup NB, Flor H, Gibson S, Keefe F, Mogil JS, Ringkamp M, Sluka KA, Stevens B, Sullivan M, Tutelman P, Ushida T, Vader T. The revised IASP definition of pain: concepts, challenges, and compromise. Pain. 2020;161(9):1976–82. https://doi.org/10.1097/j.pain.0000000000001939.
Smith B, Ceusters W, Goldberg LJ, Ohrbach RK. Towards an ontology of pain and pain-related phenomena. In: Okada M, editor. Proceedings of the conference on ontology and analytical metaphysics. Tokyo: Keio University Press; 2011. p. 23–36.
Sternbach RA. Pain: a psychophysiological analysis. New York: Academic Press; 1968.
Treede R-D. The International Association for the Study of Pain definition of pain: as valid in 2018 as in 1979, but in need of regularly updated footnotes. Pain Rep. 2018;3:e643. https://doi.org/10.1097/PR9.0000000000000643.
Weisman A, Quintner J, Cohen M. Adieu to an aphorism: why nociception is necessary for pain. Brain. 2026;149(2):422–31. https://doi.org/10.1093/brain/awaf387.
Williams AC, Craig KD. Updating the definition of pain. Pain. 2016;157:2420–3. https://doi.org/10.1097/j.pain.0000000000000613.
Wright A. A criticism of the IASP'S definition of pain. J Conscious Stud. 2011;18:19–44.

Chronic Pain: A Study in Language and Meaning

Abstract In the recent 11th revision of the International Classification of Diseases (ICD-11), chronic pain, defined as pain that has persisted for 3 months, is accorded an entry as a taxonomic entity and therefore as a *de facto* diagnostic label in its own right. While this is a welcome development towards the recognition of chronic pain as a societal problem, with potentially positive administrative applications, the question arises of whether this "entity" carries clinical meaning.

The approach taken in this Chapter is to pose a series of questions that challenge current usage of language in clinical contexts. Specifically, is "chronic pain":

- a "disorder"; if so, what is its nature?
- a disease; if so, what is its pathology?
- a symptom; if so, of what?
- an agent, a cause or a "thing"; if so, what does "it" do?
- a diagnosis; if so, what meaning does it convey to either the experiencer or the observer?

It is argued that while pain itself is denoted as being linked to tissue damage, there can be no satisfactory understanding of "chronic pain" for those who have that experience. Thus, an impasse has been reached. Although chronic pain is now appreciated clinically through a socio-psycho-biological framework, a satisfactory and concise diagnostic formulation to embrace these three dimensions has not yet been devised. As such, the meaning of chronic pain remains elusive. This has implications for validation of the perspectives of both pain experiencers and pain observers.

In chapter "Trying to Gain Traction on a Slippery Subject", pain was presented as an aporia, with the uncertainty, imprecision and intangibility that are entailed. Nonetheless, we are constrained to use language to express, describe and try to explain the experience of pain, especially in a clinical context. In chapter "Clarifying

M. Cohen, J. Quintner, *A Philosophical Handbook for Pain Medicine Practice*,
https://doi.org/10.1007/978-981-92-1682-6_3

the Definition of Pain", the vexed issue of how to define pain was addressed, with a proposed set of solutions that seek to remove ambiguity and promote clarity. Realistically, however, it will take some time for those proposals to be formally addressed in the pain community. There remains a challenge to deal with other concepts in the current pain vocabulary, in particular that of "chronic pain".

"Chronic" has only one denotation, namely a defined duration, but quite a different connotation, of being unrelated to an underlying biomedical disease process.

"Acute" vs "Chronic" Pain

"Acute" pain does not pose the divergence between denotation and connotation mentioned above. Firstly, "acute" means of short duration and, secondly, that experience is most commonly associated with active tissue damage[1] (even if a contingent association with nociception is preferred).

Indeed that is the essence of the IASP definition of pain in both its iterations. For the moment, let the 2020 iteration of the IASP definition of pain (Raja et al. 2020), be whittled down from

> an unpleasant sensory and emotional experience associated with, or resembling that associated with, actual or potential tissue damage

to

> an experience associated with tissue damage.

There can be no doubt that a human condition[2] called "chronic pain" exists. From the whittled-down definition above, it denotes "a chronic experience associated with tissue damage". Historically, chronic pain has been variously conceptualised as pain lasting or recurring for more than 3–6 months (Merskey and Bogduk 1994) or as that which persists past normal healing time (Bonica 1953). An implicit presumption of the latter conception is that an "injury"—or episode of acute tissue damage—is a necessary prerequisite for chronic pain (as actually enshrined in the fundamental IASP definition). Any temporal qualifier of "pain", such as "chronic", cannot do other than perpetuate that fundamental definition including the link with tissue damage. The question arises, is this definitional link valid?

---

[1] A less common usage of "acute" pain is an exacerbation—that is, an increase in intensity—of pain in the context of a chronic or persistent pain experience. When that context is pain secondary to a disease process, such as arthritis or cancer or the effects of chemotherapy, the pain-tissue damage nexus is not challenged. The problem occurs when the chronic or persistent pain experience is not readily attributable to a disease process, as codified in ICD-11 by "chronic primary pain". However, both these "primary" and "secondary" situations gloss over an acute-on-chronic pain experience that may be unrelated to "tissue damage". See chapter "Clarifying the Definition of Pain".

[2] "Condition" is a general term that refers to an overall state of health.

In the recent 11th revision of the International Classification of Diseases (ICD-11), chronic pain, defined as pain that has persisted for 3 months, is accorded an entry as a taxonomic entity and therefore as a *de facto* diagnostic label in its own right. This may be of use for administrative purposes such as coding, bureaucratic validation and epidemiological research. However, the approach taken here is to pose a series of questions that challenge current usage of this term in the clinical context.

Is "chronic pain":

- a "disorder"; if so, what is its nature?
- a disease; if so, what is its pathology?
- a symptom; if so, of what?
- an agent, a cause or a "thing"; if so, what does "it" do?
- a diagnosis; if so, what meaning does it convey to the experiencer or to the observer?

Before tackling these questions, it is necessary to briefly address the issues of language and meaning.

Language and Meaning in Pain Medicine

Language is the medium of conferring meaning. This speaks to the importance of communication between patient and clinician, where difficulties can arise due to the discordance between the personal experience of illness and its scientific understanding, and to the impossibility of defining a limit as to what should be communicated (Tallis 2004).

Medical language plays a strong role in the description of illness: a simple change in terminology can result in different interpretations of a known condition in terms of its seriousness and potential implications (Young et al. 2007), while vagueness in terminology in situations of uncertainty can amplify patient distress (Peters et al. 2017).

Underlying this conundrum is the issue of "meaning", a word that challenges itself. Two broad types of meaning have been identified: denotative, which refers to how a word, a sign, a symbol or a sentence is to be decoded; and existential, which refers to meanings of life or for living (Baumeister and Landau 2018). Even in this discussion, which is limited to the denotative meaning of the word "pain", some symbols have different meanings depending on the context, and "pain" is one such symbol.

To quote Baumeister and Landau (2018):

> … symbols point to other symbols in networks, indeed ones that require a *community of brains that can create shared understandings*. The connections that constitute those networks are social conventions, laws and the like. Hence a symbol's meaning inheres in its position within a network rather than its resemblance to physical things. (p. 2; emphasis added here)

To paraphrase these authors' next sentence, the meaning of "pain" within a network of symbols is independent of any specific physical facts (such as nociception, neural pathways or brain activation).

In the current discussion, the main "symbols" are words. It has long been appreciated that the meaning of language is not to be found in dictionaries, which consist of a list of substituted symbols: "This can be substituted for that in such and such circumstances" (Ogden and Richards 1946:207). However, formal attempts to define the term "meaning" have resulted in confusion, as evidenced by a "widely divergent set of opinions in the writings of the best philosophers" (Ogden and Richards 1946:248).

Although it has been suggested that humans are motivated to share thoughts and ideas with others, and that people use meaning through the vehicle of language to connect socially with other people, the question of what linguistic symbols actually mean needs to be further explored. This has been referred to as the "aboutness" of language by contemporary philosopher Horst Ruthrof (2011:89).

Philosopher Ludwig Wittgenstein (2009:§43) took a bold step by defining the meaning of a word as the way it is used in the language. In his earlier work, he had conceived of language as mediating between thought and the reality that it is about. However, in his later work, Wittgenstein moved away from seeing meanings as mental states—pictures, descriptions or images of thoughts, objects or actions "in the mind"—but rather as being enshrined in the words themselves that are being used, that are always linked to personal experiences as actions and outcomes involved in social practices:

> When I think in language, there aren't "meanings" going through my mind in addition to the verbal expressions; the language is itself the vehicle of thought. (Wittgenstein 2009:§329)

That is to say, Wittgenstein demoted imagination or mental projection of relevant scenarios as a fundamental ingredient of language to a role only auxiliary to usage in generating meaning.

However, Ruthrof (2011) argues that this highly influential definition of linguistic meaning as "use" can be only a partial account of what actually occurs. He deprecates Wittgenstein's demotion in importance of mental states such as imagination (German: *Vorstellung*), citing his reference to "image-mongery" (*Vorstellerei*), which "is of no interest to us" (Wittgenstein 2009:§390).

By contrast, Ruthrof (2000) points to the utility of phrases such as "We can imagine…", "It is easy to imagine…", "Think how…" or "Suppose…". Thus, Ruthrof attempts to meld Wittgenstein's insistence on let the use teach you the meaning with a promotion of *Vorstellung* back to being an important ingredient of language:

> If you are able to imagine what I am talking about and the way I am saying it, then there is meaning; if not, there is not. And vice versa, if I am able to imagine what others are talking about and the way they do so, an event of linguistic meaning has occurred: if not, it has not. (Ruthrof 2014:1)

It follows that in order to use language meaningfully, "members of a speech community must be able to share, to a high degree, the way in which language and nonverbal readings are to be associated with one another" (Jackendoff 2012:vi). Nonverbal readings include the activation of linguistic expressions by various stimuli—visual, aural, tactile, olfactory, gustatory—such as eye contact, tone of voice, facial expression, gestures and body posture, collectively known as "body language", itself a set of symbols that also reflect social conventions.

When concluding his detailed exegesis of Wittgenstein's approach, Ruthrof (2011) suggests "...the search for meaning in interpretive use of language turns out to be a search for what language is about, or its extensional connection. What is at stake in defining meaning as 'use' is the process between language and its aboutness" (p. 89). In this view, language, especially if novel, acts as a set of instructions for exploring pathways towards different possible meanings, and is therefore an important tool (instrument) to negotiate meanings in everyday discourse (Ruthrof 2000).

From this analysis, which recalls the importance of context and "a community of brains" as quoted above, it might be concluded that determining meaning in a clinical context is also *ultimately subject to negotiation between patient and clinician.* This is especially so with a pain experience, which can be communicated only through metaphor and simile, as well as by "body language". Provided both parties are familiar with the same community sanctioned figures of speech or symbols, they may agree upon a common meaning.

Ruthrof (2014) introduced the term "sufficient semiosis" when referring to the situation when there is community agreement on common ground for communication to take place. It explains how ordinary communication is possible without needing to invoke truth:

> Sufficient semiosis is the principle of a chain of mental representations and reasoning in support of synthetic judgments. The point at which such a chain is regarded as sufficient is determined not logically but only pragmatically, when a community is satisfied that the judgment is well grounded in shared social experience. (Ruthrof 2014:49)

Denotations of Chronic Pain

Is "Chronic Pain" a Disorder?

A "disorder" in the health context generally refers to a specific disturbance or abnormality of body function, physiological or psychological. That raises the question of whether "pain" is an abnormal phenomenon or, as discussed in chapter "The Salient Role of Nociception", an evolutionarily conserved normal event. *Chronic* pain presents an apparent paradox between being considered maladaptive (from the human perspective) yet associated with possible survival value over evolution. That very statement risks confusing pain with nociception, when it is the latter that is the survival mechanism. However, to the extent that the chronic pain experience may reflect sensitised nociception, which in turn would be a "disturbance" of normal body function, it seems reasonable that it could be considered a "disorder".

Is "Chronic Pain" a Symptom?

The term "symptom" is derived from the Greek expression *sumptoma* (συμπτώμα), conceptualised as an occurrence or happening, but also as an implied prediction or portent as to what might befall that person (Temkin 1977). Symptoms are experiential reports presented to the clinician by the patient in the course of the medical consultation (King 1982; Nessa 1996). As undeniable "natural facts", symptoms constitute core components of the diagnostic process (Eriksen and Risør 2013) and can be regarded as cultural and communicative acts. In this case, they can be seen as an attempt by the patient to enable the clinician to experience something akin to their own experience (Semino 2010), which is the essence of empathy (Stein 1989).[3]

However, as symptoms may be impossible to convey by literal language, they are frequently expressed as metaphors or similes. Metaphors for pain include such descriptors as "cutting", "burning", "stabbing" and "piercing". Common similes that are used include chest pain described as like "a band or tightness around the chest", headache as "a pounding within my skull" and abdominal pain as "something is gripping me". The clinician is then charged with the responsibility of trying to understand the meaning of the symptom when thus conveyed (Periyakoil 2008). In a multi-cultural context, the potential for misunderstanding complicates this responsibility (Masukume and Zumla 2012).

Traditionally, symptoms have been interpreted as indicators of disease. As will be discussed in chapter "The Non-Convergent Language Used in Clinical and Taxonomic Settings", the taxonomy of ICD-11 has elevated "chronic secondary pain" to a clinical problem in its own right, as well as being a symptom of an underlying disease process. However, that interpretation is challenged when there is no evidence of underlying disease, as in "chronic primary pain". Clearly, "chronic pain" cannot be a symptom of itself, so from the point of view of the experiencer, there is no fixed framework of reference—or denotation—that might facilitate communication.

Is Chronic Pain a Disease?

Chronic pain has been framed as a distinct medical condition. Bonica (1976) regarded intractable pain as "a destructive force that often imposes severe emotional, physical, economic, and sociological stresses on the patient as well as his

---

[3] Empathy is discussed in chapter "The Clinical (Two-Person) Encounter".

family as well as on society". Other conceptualisations of chronic pain have included "pain without apparent biological value", which contains a teleological if not also moral judgment, and "persistent pain that is as a rule not amenable to treatments based upon specific remedies" (Merskey and Bogduk 1994), which begs the question of "specific remedies" and almost justifies therapeutic nihilism.

These arguments signalled a major conceptual shift in pain medicine, from viewing chronic pain as a presenting symptom of disease to an entity-in-itself or a physical "thing" possessing agency; that is, an instrument able to exert causal power or elicit other effects. There is a tension therefore between the pain experience, which is not a "thing" as discussed in chapter "Trying to Gain Traction on a Slippery Subject", and pain conceptualised in clinical medicine as a disease, which clearly is a "thing" (Quintner et al. 2008). Dorland's Illustrated Medical Dictionary (2007), offers this definition of disease: "any deviation from or interruption of the normal structure or function of any body part, organ, or system that is manifested by a characteristic set of symptoms and signs and whose aetiology, pathology, and prognosis may be known or unknown".

Despite the insistence on the presence of "a characteristic set of symptoms and signs", this and similar dictionary denotations fail to convey that the concept of "any deviation from or interruption of the normal structure or function of any body part, organ, or system" is in fact a high-level abstraction or stipulation that is largely consensus-driven within the medical community (Rosenberg 2002; Body and Foex 2009). In this light, those who argue that chronic pain is a disease in its own right seek to superimpose a well-trodden map of biomedicine over a conceptually complex landscape, which is experienced, lived and felt by the person experiencing pain (Cohen et al. 2013). A contemporary example of imposing a "biomedical consensus" is the condition labelled as "myofascial pain", which is used as a surrogate for an as yet unknown but presumed disease process[4] (Quintner et al. 2015).

The proposition by Siddall and Cousins (2004) of pain-as-a-disease arose out of their dissatisfaction with pain being classed only as a nonspecific symptom of disease, taken together with an undue deference being paid to the biomedical imperative to identify and treat any underlying disease. Having reviewed the evidence to date on the physiology of nociception and how that might be perturbed, they concluded: "Persistent pain has its own pathology, symptoms and signs and is therefore a disease entity". However, this assertion raises the question, which "characteristic" clinical features apart from the complaint of pain constitute the "disease" of pain (Cohen et al. 2013)? Here it is argued that, for chronic pain to be considered a disease, "it is not sufficient to invoke a syndrome or a grouping of symptoms of which pain might be a component, especially when the diversity of conditions associated with pain is considered" (p. 1287). In conclusion, on neither pathological nor clinical criteria can pain-as-a-disease be justified.

---

[4] See chapter "Case Studies in Tautology, Circular Reasoning and Conflation: Fibromyalgia and Myofascial Pain "Syndromes" for discussion of "myofascial pain".

Is Chronic Pain a Diagnosis?

If chronic pain is not a disease, can it nonetheless be denoted as a diagnosis? Ever since the emergence of Medicine as a scientific discipline in Ancient Greece, diagnosis has played a pivotal role (Kleisiaris et al. 2014). In modern times, diagnosis has become inextricably related to specific disease formulations that serve simultaneously to legitimise both the patient's experience and the physician's status in society as a healer (Crookshank 1946). Diagnosis, from the Greek dia (διά-) denoting "through" and gnosis (-γνωσις), denoting "knowledge", originally referred to the *process* of identifying in the body underlying causal associations considered responsible for the patient's complaints and then conferring an "appropriate" label (Bichat 1825). In its simplest form, medical diagnosis consists of linking symptoms reported by the patient and a lesion observed in the tissue (the clinicopathologic inference) (Bichat 1825).

In addition to identifying the steps to be taken for such identification, diagnosis has become connoted as implying deeper inherent knowledge, if not also certainty (Cohen et al. 2013). Even though they lack definite physical properties (mass, velocity, chemical composition, etc.) and therefore are detached from the physical world of things, medical diagnoses can exert real effects on that world through their meaning to the patient within the structure of a society because of the value judgments implicit within them (Barraclough 2004). For example, whereas some soldiers from the Boer War were seen as "cowards", those from the First World War with similar symptoms had "shell shock" or conversion hysteria and those from the Vietnam War had post-traumatic stress disorder (PTSD) (Summerfield 2001) reflecting a change from a derogatory label to a medically acceptable one.

Medical diagnoses tend to be concrete concepts, simultaneously implying understanding of a condition and the therapeutic pathway to be followed. Diagnostic labels thus not only become facts (or "things") in the real world but also form the basis for ways of structuring reality through particular interpretations, conjectures and hypotheses. The knowledge implied by a diagnostic label is utilised in two ways. Firstly, it provides a potential source of meaning for the patient and thus the basis for narratives and stories that will have meaning to others whose voices also need to be heard and acknowledged, such as family members, society, ethicists, insurance companies and others (Hanne 2015). As expressed by Jutel (2009:942):

> From the patient's perspective, the diagnosis and the metaphors employed to explain that diagnosis should clarify the patient's story of symptoms and help to render his or her experiential world comprehensible.

Secondly, by structuring the approach of the physician to the problem, the knowledge implicit in the diagnostic label "underlies the socially indispensable tasks of diagnosis and prognosis and the rationalization of therapeutic practice" (Body and Foex 2009). But do these principles apply to chronic pain? Does any denotation of the term "clarify the patient's story" or, for that matter, "help to render … comprehensible" the world of the patient or of the physician? And does that term introduce rational therapy?

Following the rules or procedures for making a diagnosis, as laid out by Bowen (2006), chronic pain would form part of the process of data collection, but illness scripts would default to those associated with tissue damage, according to the IASP definition of pain.

An Impasse?

To return to the original questions proposed above:

- Is chronic pain a "disorder"? Yes, in which the disturbance of function relates to nociception.
- Is chronic pain a "disease"? No, as characteristic clinical features cannot be identified.
- Is chronic pain a "symptom"? Yes, but there is no consensus on "of what".
- Is chronic pain a "diagnosis"? No, as it provides neither clarity nor therapeutic pathway to either experiencer or clinician.
- Is chronic pain an "agent", a "cause" or a "thing"? Not as a material entity that has agency but possibly as a process that does so.[5]

In fact, it may be concluded that a paradox has been reached, in which chronic pain itself is conceptualised as an experience but not a physical "thing", while the use of that same term as a diagnostic label, which is a "thing" that has agentive properties, identifies only one interpretation, which does not capture that experience. This construal implies that to be diagnosed with "chronic pain" may in fact not be meaningful to the person with that experience.

Why has Ruthrof's "sufficient semiosis" been so elusive here? If language can achieve meaning through use and imaginability, why have these terms failed to imply agreement within a language community? "Disease" and "diagnosis" may well work for the discourse between pain observers but not for experiencers, for whom "disorder" and "symptom" seem self-evident. For them, promoting chronic pain as a disease or a diagnosis fails to capture denotational meaning let alone existential meaning which, as suggested by Baumeister and Landau (2018), involves purpose, value, mattering, continuity and coherence.

This analysis of whether "chronic pain" has meaning has in fact exposed the conjunction of two imponderables: the meaning of "meaning" and the "aporia" of pain.[6] In seeking to limit "meaning" to its denotative (or definitional) usage, any argument is constrained by the definitional linkage of "pain" to tissue damage, which presents the problem of finding the words to describe the experience when tissue damage is unknown or unknowable. Another constraint is the differing

---

[5] See chapter "Trying to Gain Traction on a Slippery Subject".

[6] As discussed in chapter "Trying to Gain Traction on a Slippery Subject".

perspectives of the pain experiencer and the pain observer,[7] especially when both parties reside in "a community of brains that can create shared understandings".[8]

It does seem that an impasse has been reached. Although chronic pain is now appreciated through a socio-psycho-biological framework[9] (Carr and Bradshaw 2014), a satisfactory and concise diagnostic formulation to embrace these three dimensions has not yet been devised.[10] Most conditions refracted through the medical lens tend to be classified in terms of disturbed anatomy and/or physiology and/or biochemistry, to the exclusion of psychological, social and cultural factors. Because pain is experienced in the body, its description, discussion and classification have tended to be expressed in somatic terminologies in accordance with the clinicopathological method (Sullivan 1998).

Thus, the impasse may be the definition itself of pain. It follows that resolution of this impasse may lie in a thorough re-examination of that definition, as was discussed in chapter "Clarifying the Definition of Pain".

References

Barraclough K. Diagnosis and Wittgenstein's theories of language. Br J Gen Pract. 2004;54(503):480–1.

Baumeister RE, Landau MJ. Finding the meaning of meaning: emerging insights from four grand questions. Rev Gen Psychol. 2018;22(1):1–10. https://doi.org/10.1037/gpr0000145.

Bichat X. Anatomie générale appliquée à la physiologie et à medicine, vol. 3. Paris: Broson, Gabon et Cie; 1825.

Body R, Foex B. On the philosophy of diagnosis: is doing more good than harm better than "primum non nocere"? Emerg Med J. 2009;26:238–40. https://doi.org/10.1136/emj.2008.064303.

Bonica JJ. The management of pain. Philadelphia: Lea and Febiger; 1953.

Bonica JJ. Introduction to the first world congress on pain. In: Bonica JJ, Albe-Fessard DG, editors. Advances in pain research and therapy, vol. 1. New York: Raven Press; 1976. p. xxvii–xxix.

Bowen JL. Educational strategies to promote clinical diagnostic reasoning. New Engl J Med. 2006;355:2217–25. https://doi.org/10.1056/NEJMra054782.

Carr DB, Bradshaw YS. Time to flip the pain curriculum? Anesthesiology. 2014;120:12–4. https://doi.org/10.1097/ALN.0000000000000054.

Cohen ML, Quintner JL, Buchanan DA. Is chronic pain a disease? Pain Med. 2013;14:1284–8. https://doi.org/10.1111/pme.12025.

Crookshank FG. The importance of a theory of signs and a critique of language in the study of medicine. In: Ogden CK, Richards IA, editors. The meaning of meaning. 8th ed. New York: Harcourt, Brace and World, Inc.; 1946. p. 337–55.

Eriksen TE, Risør MB. What is called symptom? Med Health Care Philos. 2013;17(1):89–102. https://doi.org/10.1007/s11019-013-9501-5.10.1007/s11019-012-9346-2.

[7] These differing perspectives were discussed in chapter "Clarifying the Definition of Pain".

[8] Ways of understanding how these two parties interact in the cinical encounter are discussed in chapter "The Clinical (Two-Person) Encounter".

[9] This is addressed in detail in chapter "Conceptual Frameworks".

[10] This is discussed in chapter "Translation into the Clinic".

Hanne M. Diagnosis and metaphor. Perspect Biol Med. 2015;58:35–52. https://doi.org/10.1353/pbm.2015.0010.
Jackendoff R. A user's guide to thought and meaning. Oxford: Oxford University Press; 2012.
Jutel A. Sociology of diagnosis: a preliminary review. Sociol Health Illn. 2009;31:278–99. https://doi.org/10.1111/j.1467-9566.2008.01152.x.
King LS. Medical thinking: a historical preface. Princeton: Princeton University Press; 1982. p. 91–104.
Kleisiaris CF, Sfakianakis C, Papathanasious IV. Health care practices in ancient Greece: the Hippocratic ideal. J Med Ethics Hist Med. 2014;7:6. eCollection 2014
Masukume G, Zumla A. Analogies and metaphors in clinical medicine. Clin Med. 2012;12:55–6. https://doi.org/10.7861/clinmedicine.12-1-55.
Merskey H, Bogduk N, editors. Classification of chronic pain: descriptions of chronic pain syndromes and definition of pain terms. 2nd ed. Seattle: IASP Press; 1994.
Nessa J. About signs and symptoms: can semiotics expand the view of clinical medicine? Theor Med. 1996;17:363–77. https://doi.org/10.1007/BF004896.
Ogden CK, Richards IA, editors. The meaning of meaning. 8th ed. New York: Harcourt, Brace and World, Inc.; 1946.
Periyakoil VS. Using metaphors in medicine. J Palliat Care. 2008;11(6):842–4. https://doi.org/10.1089/jpm.2008.9885.
Peters A, McEwan BS, Friston K. Uncertainty and stress: why it causes diseases and how it is mastered by the brain. Prog Neurobiol. 2017;156:164–88. https://doi.org/10.1016/j.pneurobio.2017.05.004.
Quintner JL, Buchanan D, Cohen ML, Katz J, Williamson O. Pain medicine and its models: helping or hindering? Pain Med. 2008;9:824–34. https://doi.org/10.1111/j.1526-4637.2007.00391.x.
Quintner J, Bove G, Cohen M. A critical evaluation of the "trigger point" phenomenon. Rheumatology. 2015;54:392–39. https://doi.org/10.1093/rheumatology/keu471.
Raja SN, Carr DB, Cohen M, Finnerup NB, Flor H, Gibson S, Keefe F, Mogil JS, Ringkamp M, Sluka KA, Stevens B, Sullivan M, Tutelman P, Ushida T, Vader T. The revised IASP definition of pain: concepts, challenges, and compromise. Pain. 2020;161(9):1976–82. https://doi.org/10.1097/j.pain.0000000000001939.
Rosenberg CE. The tyranny of diagnosis: specific entities and individual experience. Milbank Q. 2002;80:237–60. https://doi.org/10.1111/1468-0009.t01-1-00003.
Ruthrof H. The body in language. London: Cassell; 2000. p. vii.
Ruthrof H. Language, *Vorstellung*, and meaning as use. Linguist Philos Investig. 2011;10:60–92.
Ruthrof H. Language and imaginability. Newcastle Upon Tyne: Cambridge Scholar Publishing; 2014. https://doi.org/10.5840/ajs2015311/24.
Saunders W. Dorland's illustrated medical dictionary. 31st ed. Philadelphia: Saunders; 2007.
Semino E. Descriptions of pain, metaphor and embodied simulation. Metaphor Symb. 2010;25(4):205–26. https://doi.org/10.1080/10926488.2010.510926.
Siddall PJ, Cousins MJ. Persistent pain as a disease entity: implications for clinical management. Anesth Analg. 2004;99:510–20. https://doi.org/10.1213/01.ANE.0000133383.17666.3A.
Stein E. On the problem of empathy. Stein W, transl. Washington: ICS Publications; 1989.
Sullivan M. The problem of pain in the clinicopathological method. Clin J Pain. 1998;14(3):197–20. https://doi.org/10.1097/00002508-199809000-00005.
Summerfield D. The invention of post-traumatic stress disorder and the social usefulness of a psychiatric category. BMJ. 2001;322:95–8. https://doi.org/10.1136/bmj.322.7278.95.
Tallis R. Hippocratic oaths: medicine and its discontents. London: Atlantic Books; 2004. p. 43–73.
Temkin O. The double face of Janus. Baltimore: The Johns Hopkins University Press; 1977. p. 419–40.

Wittgenstein L. Philosophical investigations. Translated by GEM Anscombe, PMS Hacker & Joachim Schulte. Oxford: Blackwell; 2009.

Young ME, Brookes L, Norman GR. Found in translation: the impact of familiar symptom descriptions on diagnosis in novices. Med Educ. 2007;14:1146–51. https://doi.org/10.1111/j.1365-2923.2007.02913.x.

The Non-Convergent Language Used in Clinical and Taxonomic Settings

Abstract The incorporation of "chronic pain" as a taxonomic entity into ICD-11 has been of major benefit towards the recognition of that human experience at epidemiological and administrative, if not also political, levels. This incorporation occurred in parallel with the 2020 revision of the IASP definition of pain which, as discussed in chapter "Clarifying the Definition of Pain", does not resolve significant ambiguities. In chapter "Chronic Pain: A Study in Language and Meaning", it was argued that the term "chronic pain" does not convey meaning for experiencers. This chapter addresses the question of whether, despite those two caveats, that development also has clinical utility.

The ICD-11 classification identified six pragmatic clusters of chronic "secondary" pain for those instances in which pain is attributable to another condition, which logically left a seventh category of chronic "primary" pain, which essentially is any pain that is not considered to be "secondary". However, chronic "primary" pain has become stranded, as that label does not add meaning for the pain experiencer and also is of little help to clinicians in terms of attempting to apply a systematic approach to the diagnosis and management of their patients' predicaments.

In parallel with—but isolated from—this incorporation was the development of the construct of "nociplastic pain", which has become conflated with the stranded chronic "primary" pain, even though "nociplastic", once validated, would fall under the "secondary" category of the ICD-11 taxonomy. Taken together with the differing principles on which the "secondary" chronic pain categories were constructed, this conflation questions the utility of "secondary" as well as "primary" chronic pain as clinical labels.

In chapter "Clarifying the Definition of Pain", the challenges of defining "pain" for the purposes of enquiry, especially scientific and clinical, were addressed. That chapter concluded by suggesting that a definition of pain should distinguish that experience from nociception on the one hand and from suffering on the other. The

M. Cohen, J. Quintner, *A Philosophical Handbook for Pain Medicine Practice*,
https://doi.org/10.1007/978-981-92-1682-6_4

suggested changes maintain the intent of the current definitions but remove ambiguity and provide clarity.

In chapter "Chronic Pain: A Study in Language and Meaning", another source of confusion was examined, namely the connotation of the qualifier "chronic" in "chronic pain", where "pain" still depends on the current definition (Raja et al. 2020). It was argued that to be labelled as having "chronic pain" may not be meaningful to the person with that experience. Just as "pain" is not a diagnosis, neither is "chronic pain" a useful clinical concept.

Nonetheless, in 2022, the term "chronic pain" was introduced as a *taxonomic* entity into the International Classification of Diseases (ICD-11). While this has been a welcome development in terms of recognition of that disorder—as a "condition-in-its-own-right"—for administrative and epidemiological purposes, there are questions regarding its clinical utility which this chapter will address.

Incorporation of "Chronic Pain" into ICD-11

As discussed in chapter "Clarifying the Definition of Pain", the intention of the 1979 definition of pain was to be a taxonomic exercise. However, it became clear that, as a definition, it did not demarcate pain from non-pain but rather was an operational term for clinical practice (Wright 2017).

In parallel with the process of revision of the IASP definition of pain (2018–2020) (Raja et al. 2020) was the work of the joint Task Force of the IASP and the World Health Organisation (WHO) (2012–2019) towards incorporating pain as a condition in its own right into the 11th Revision of the International Classification of Diseases (ICD-11) (Treede et al. 2019). For this purpose, the 1979 iteration of the IASP definition was used.

In ICD-11, which was promulgated in 2022, chronic pain, defined as pain that has persisted for 3 months, is accorded an entry as a *taxonomic* entity and therefore as a *de facto* potential diagnostic label in its own right. In developing this classification of chronic pain as an identifiable condition,[1] the joint IASP/WHO Task Force allocated the many and diverse examples of that condition into seven subcategories (Treede et al. 2019).

In accordance with WHO criteria, the Task Force attempted to give first priority to aetiology of pain, followed by underlying pathophysiological mechanism, and finally the body site in which pain is experienced. Also employed was the WHO principle of "multiple parenting", which allows any one example to be included under more than one category. This was appropriate as clinically, even when clearly associated with another diagnosis, the chronic pain experience itself can be as much

[1] The Task Force (and its publications) used "condition". In view of the discussion in chapter "Chronic Pain: A Study in Language and Meaning", "disorder" would have been more appropriate.

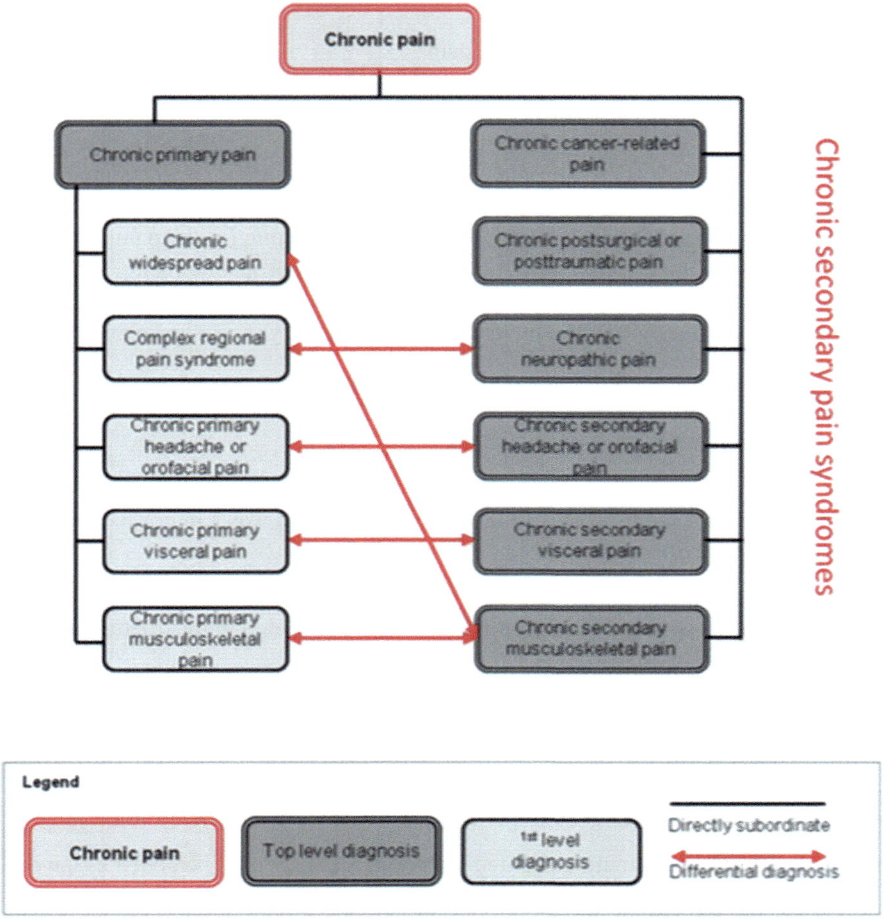

Fig. 1 Structure of the IASP classification of chronic pain. (Reproduced with permission from Treede et al. (2019:21))

a source of suffering and of therapeutic challenge as any underlying disease process (Fig. 1).

The ICD-11 classification identified six pragmatic clusters of chronic "secondary" pain for those instances in which pain was attributable to another condition:

- chronic cancer-related pain
- chronic postsurgical and posttraumatic pain
- chronic neuropathic pain
- chronic secondary headache or orofacial pain

- chronic secondary visceral pain
- chronic secondary musculoskeletal pain

The pragmatism of these clusters relates to the principles on which they were constructed:

- *Aetiology* with respect to chronic cancer-related and chronic post-traumatic and post-surgical pain, the implication being that the cancer (and treatment thereof) or surgery or trauma respectively are directly responsible for the pain[2]
- *Mechanism of nociception* with respect to chronic neuropathic pain
- *Body site of pain* with respect to chronic secondary headache or orofacial pain, chronic secondary visceral pain and chronic secondary musculoskeletal pain

In taxonomic usage, this concept of "secondary" allows co-coding of a patient's pain as a condition-in-its-own-right along with the underlying disease to which the pain is attributable.

For examples:

- a patient with osteoarthrosis of the knee in whom pain was a major factor would be coded as having
  - (i) knee osteoarthrosis
    (ii) chronic secondary musculoskeletal pain associated with structural change (ICD-11 code: MG30.31)
- a patient with pain attributed to diabetic polyneuropathy would be coded as having
  - (i) diabetic polyneuropathy
    (ii) chronic peripheral neuropathic pain[3] (ICD-11 code: MG30.51)
- a patient with pelvic pain attributed to endometriosis would be coded as having
  - (i) endometriosis
    (ii) chronic secondary visceral pain from persistent inflammation (ICD-11 code: MG30.42)

This process exposed the challenge of categorising chronic pain that cannot be associated with or attributed to another condition, thereby logically attracting the label "chronic primary pain", which was defined as:

> … chronic pain in one or more anatomic regions that persists or recurs for longer than 3 months and is associated with significant emotional distress (e.g., anxiety, anger, frustration, or depressed mood) and/or significant functional disability (interference in activities of daily life and participation in social roles) and that cannot be better accounted for by another chronic pain condition. (Nicholas et al. 2019)

[2] To avoid the *post hoc ergo propter hoc* fallacy.

[3] "Neuropathic" pain is by definition "secondary".

In stark contrast, however, to the entities subsumed under "chronic secondary pain", in which the label "chronic pain" is comorbid with another diagnosis, the label "chronic primary pain" promotes the symptom itself to the level of a condition in its own right and therefore as a diagnostic entity. This blurring between symptom, condition and diagnosis means in effect that a patient presenting with "chronic pain" is diagnosed as having a condition called "chronic pain" which is then coded for epidemiological and administrative purposes as "chronic primary pain".

The denotation of "chronic primary pain" in fact comprises four elements:

(i) pain: the experience is or is considered to be associated with tissue damage
(ii) chronic: the experience has persisted for 3 months
(iii) primary: the experience "cannot be better accounted for by another chronic pain condition"
(iv) the experience is "associated with significant emotional distress and/or significant functional disability"

As element (iv) also occurs in instances of "chronic secondary pain", the pathognomonic feature of "chronic primary pain" is element (iii)—"cannot be better accounted for by another chronic pain condition". This can be seen also to be fundamentally constrained by the denotational link of "pain" to "tissue damage", as discussed in chapter "Clarifying the Definition of Pain".

This is by no means an argument against the inclusion of "pain" and "chronic pain" in ICD-11, which has been a necessary and a welcome development towards the recognition of chronic pain as a societal and clinical problem, with positive administrative implications and the *possibility* of positive diagnostic and therapeutic consequences.

However, it does leave "chronic primary pain" stranded, as that label is devoid of meaning for the pain experiencer (as discussed in chapter "Chronic Pain: A Study in Language and Meaning") and also is of little utility for clinicians attempting to apply a systematic approach to the diagnosis and management of their patients' predicaments.

Conflation of Non-Convergent Terms

The question now arises, what effect does ICD-11 labelling have in the clinic?

To take one of the examples above of dual "taxonomic" labelling in the cases of chronic *secondary* pain:

- a patient with pelvic pain attributed to endometriosis would be coded as having
  - *endometriosis* and
    chronic secondary visceral pain from persistent *inflammation*

This is in fact triple labelling with (a) a *pathological* label, "endometriosis"; (b) a *taxonomic* (ICD-11) label, "chronic secondary visceral pain"; and (c) a *mechanistic* label, "inflammation". This last label, (c), although speculative, is in effect a hypothesis of nociception, where "nociception" refers to activation of the nociceptive apparatus. Currently, this example would attract the so-called "descriptor" of "nociceptive pain", although that is a misnomer.[4]

The above labelling then becomes:

- endometriosis (underlying pathological process)
- chronic secondary visceral pain (ICD-11)
- "nociceptive" nociception[5]

Such triple labelling may well provide a comprehensive description of the somatic contribution to that patient's pain, although it could be argued that the second dot-point is unnecessary.

This emphasises how stranded is the term "chronic primary pain" in terms of clinical diagnostic utility, as there is "no other chronic pain condition" and the mechanism of activation of the nociceptive apparatus is unknown. Thus, although "chronic primary pain" does serve to legitimise the predicament of many patients whose pain experience might otherwise be dismissed, it denotes only "pain of unknown pathogenesis", which may still invite stigmatisation.[6]

During the same decade (2012–2022) of the development of ICD-11 and the revision of the IASP definition of pain, there was another major conceptual initiative (2016–2017), namely the addition of the construct of "nociplastic pain" to the pre-existing "pain descriptors" ("nociceptive" and "neuropathic") (Kosek et al. 2016).

Although it was promulgated officially only in 2022, the formulation of "primary" pain in ICD-11 in fact preceded the introduction of "nociplastic pain" and is agnostic to it. Nonetheless, the assumption has been made by many authors that "primary" pain and "nociplastic" pain are synonymous, despite the first being a taxonomic concept and the second being a hypothesis of nociception. These two connotations have become confused—the differences between them have not been appreciated—and conflated—brought together as one[7] (Cohen 2022; Weisman et al. 2024; Cohen et al. 2025).

In any event, the pathognomonic criterion for "primary pain", that the pain "cannot be better accounted for by another condition", would be negated if nociplastic mechanisms, once validated, were invoked. That is, the pain would cease to be "primary" and would come under the ICD-11 secondary rubric, as "chronic secondary nociplastic pain". Taken together with the differing principles on which the

---

[4] Nociception, nociceptive apparatus and so-called "pain descriptors" are discussed in detail in chapter "The Salient Role of Nociception".

[5] See footnote 4 again.

[6] See chapter "Translation into the Clinic".

[7] A similar situation exists for the conflation between nociplastic pain and "central sensitisation of nociception". This major problem of conflation is discussed in detail in chapter "The Salient Role of Nociception".

"secondary" chronic pain categories were constructed, this questions the utility of "secondary" as well as "primary" chronic pain as clinical labels.[8]

References

Cohen ML. Clarifying "chronic primary musculoskeletal pain"? The waters remain murky. Pain Rep. 2022;7:e1021. https://doi.org/10.1097/PR9.0000000000001021.

Cohen M, Quintner J, Weisman A. "Primary" and "nociplastic" pain must not be conflated. Pain. 2025;166:1949–50. https://doi.org/10.1097/j.pain.0000000000003659.

Kosek E, Cohen M, Baron R, Gebhart GF, Mico J-A, Rice AS, Rief W, Sluka KA. Do we need a third mechanistic descriptor for chronic pain states? Pain. 2016;157:1382–6. https://doi.org/10.1097/j.pain.000000000000507.

Nicholas M, Vlaeyen JWS, Rief W, Barke A, Aziz Q, Benoliel R, Cohen M, Evers S, Giamberardino MA, Goebel A, Korwisi B, Perrot S, Svenssen P, Wang S-J, Treede R-D. IASP taskforce for the classification of chronic pain. The IASP classification of chronic pain for ICD-11: chronic primary pain. Pain. 2019;160(1):28–37. https://doi.org/10.1097/j.pain.0000000000001390.

Raja SN, Carr DB, Cohen M, Finnerup NB, Flor H, Gibson S, Keefe F, Mogil JS, Ringkam M, Sluka KA, Stevens B, Sullivan M, Tutelman P, Ushida T, Vader T. The revised IASP definition of pain: concepts, challenges, and compromise. Pain. 2020;161(9):1976–82. https://doi.org/10.1097/j.pain.0000000000001939.

Treede R-D, Rief W, Barke A, Aziz Q, Bennett MI, Benoliel R, Cohen M, Evers S, Finnerup NB, First MB, Giamberardino MA, Kaasa S, Korwisi B, Kosek E, Lavand'homme P, Nicholas M, Perrot S, Scholz J, Schug S, Sith B, Svensson P, Vlaeyen JWS, Wang S-J. Chronic pain as a symptom or a disease: the IASP classification of chronic pain for the international classification of diseases (ICD-11). Pain. 2019;160:19–27. https://doi.org/10.1097/j.pain.0000000000001384.

Weisman A, Quintner J, Cohen M. "Primary" versus "secondary" musculoskeletal pain. J Pain. 2024;25(11):104510. https://doi.org/10.1016/j.jpain.2024.03.006.

Wright A. An introduction to the IASP's definition of pain. In: Corns J, editor. The Routledge handbook of philosophy of pain. New York: Routledge; 2017. p. 367–77.

[8] This implication is discussed in chapter "Translation into the Clinic".

Conceptual Frameworks

Abstract A major change in how to conceptualise human illness occurred in 1980, when psychiatrist George Engel proposed a "biopsychosocial model" (BPS), the essence of which was that a patient's self-report of illness could be influenced and sometimes even determined not only by biological factors but also by those in the psychological, social and cultural domains. This chapter reviews the evolution of biopsychosocial approaches as applied to pain.

While of undoubted usefulness in understanding the phenomenology of pain, BPS schemata are unable to explain how the three dimensions of interest might interact. A stumbling block for BPS approaches has been their inability to transcend both biomedical reductionism and perpetuation of body-mind dualism. Thus BPS "models" are best seen as *conceptual frameworks*, offering a lens through which to see the clinical world differently, rather than describing how something "works". More recently, the BPS framework has been "inverted", to "sociopsychobiological" or "sociopsychobiomedical", to emphasise the role of non-biomedical factors.

Central to the challenge of trying to understand and thus validate the pain experience is the nature of the clinical encounter itself. A new theoretical perspective to understand this encounter draws on three vantage points:

(i) the central concept of pain as an *aporia* as discussed in chapter "Trying to Gain Traction on a Slippery Subject"; (ii) the nature of humans (and indeed other biological systems) as autonomous self-organising, self-referential, autopoietic units; and (iii) *inter-subjectivity* as the natural ground for rapprochement between the world of the clinician and the world of the person experiencing pain in the clinical setting, which will be discussed in chapter "The Clinical (Two-Person) Encounter".

M. Cohen, J. Quintner, *A Philosophical Handbook for Pain Medicine Practice*, https://doi.org/10.1007/978-981-92-1682-6_5

Models of Illness

What Are Models?

Broadly speaking, a model can be seen as an attempt to simplify a complex system. In the scientific realm, conceptual models are used to describe phenomena in order to understand and to make predictions about how something works (Gerlee and Lundh 2016:57).

When applied to scientific medicine, conceptual models are constructed from ideas and notions about mechanisms and entities within the system that is the body. They are used as learning tools or vehicles to explain and predict specific natural processes underlying bodily function (Gerlee and Lundh 2016; McLaren 1998; Radden 1999). Because they are "... simplifications of reality there are always parts of a phenomenon that a model cannot account for, or in other words there are always features of the real phenomenon that are not reflected in a single model" (Gerlee and Lundh 2016:38).

All models need to undergo regular assessment and can then be revised or, should new evidence emerge that renders them insupportable, discarded and replaced by more useful models (Reber 1985).

Biomedical Model of Illness

If illness is defined as an individual's perceived condition of poor health, then the dominant discourse in Western health care is the so-called biomedical model.

This holds that all symptoms, including pain, are expressions of a discoverable disease process and that there is a reliable connection between them (Quintner et al. 2008).

Biomedical models of disease-based illnesses originate from the German pathologist Rudolf Virchow's hypothesis that disease is the result of disturbances in the body's cellular structures (Follis 1960). But not all illness is attributable to a specific disease (Wade and Halligan 2004).

This biomedical approach is in fact an explanatory tool about how illness "works" (Quintner et al. 2008). Its effectiveness turns on the ability of the clinician to validate a patient's illness by demonstrating an underlying lesion or disease process, thus predicting its natural course and/or prescribing a program of intervention. This is achieved through a commitment to obtaining empirically observable or objective evidence, which tends to relegate behavioural, psychological and social factors to the background.

The biomedical model, as applied to pain, is depicted here:

PATHOLOGY (TISSUE DAMAGE)

↓

PAIN

Or, more correctly:

PATHOLOGY (TISSUE DAMAGE)

↓

NERVOUS SYSTEM (NOCICEPTION)

↓

PAIN

Essentially, this model posits that pain is a reliable indicator of an underlying lesion that is signalled through the nervous system; that is, a confident cause-and-effect relationship exists. The model also holds that therapeutic attention to the underlying pathology, if possible and available, should alleviate the symptoms, in this case, pain. Necessarily, this model excludes the individual's pain experience itself.

The predicament of the person experiencing chronic pain without identifiable cause and therefore without access to specific treatment then presents a conundrum, as medical practitioners struggle to validate it (Wade and Halligan 2004; Quintner et al. 2008).[1] In other words, strict application of the biomedical model denies societally determined illness status (the "sick role") being conferred upon that individual (Parsons 1951). The consequences can be denial of access to health care and denial of access to income support, as well as stigmatisation (Quintner 2020).

Biopsychosocial Frameworks of Illness

Acknowledging the benefits as well as the limitations in the application of the biomedical model of illness, psychiatrist George Engel (1980) pioneered the use of a more comprehensive schema to guide clinicians in their everyday work. Engel's approach, labelled as a "biopsychosocial (BPS) model", reflected recognition that "psychological and social factors influence a patient's perceptions and actions and therefore the experience of what it feels like to be ill" (Wade and Halligan 2004:1398). He invited clinicians to entertain the proposition that a patient's self-report of illness could be influenced and sometimes even determined not only by biological factors but also by those in the psychological, social and cultural domains.

Engel's intent was to provide a scientific framework "within which can be conceptualised and related as natural systems *all* the levels of organisation pertinent to heath and disease" (Engel 1978; emphasis added here).

Engel's BPS schema featured a hierarchically arranged continuum of systems, ranging from sub-atomic particles to the biosphere. Each system was conceptualised as being a component of higher systems in the hierarchy. Disruption of any

[1] See also chapter "Chronic Pain: A Study in Language and Meaning".

system could, at least theoretically, interfere with the functioning of other systems, and particularly of those closely situated to it in that hierarchy.

Biosychosocial Framework for Pain

Applying the systems hierarchy (left-hand column) described by Engel to pain yields broad content domains (right hand column):

Systems hierarchy level	Broad content domains
Biosphere	Philosophical issues, biological significance
Nation/society/culture	Politics, ethics, medicolegal, mythologies
Community	Economic impact, disability, handicap
Family	Sick role, illness behaviour
Two-person	Intersubjectivity
Person	Personality, self-esteem, beliefs, coping skills
Nervous system	PNS[2]/CNS,[3] nociception
Organs/organ systems	Pathology/disease
Tissues/cells	Receptors/membranes
Molecules/atoms	Neurotransmitters/cytokines

This can be distilled into three broad dimensions:

- "bio-" (for "biological"), encompassing the bottom four hierarchical levels above
- "-psycho-" (for "psychological"), accommodating the "person", "two-person" and "family" levels
- "-social", embracing the top four levels.

Engel (1980) believed his model to be scientific, as it was underpinned by General Systems Theory (GST), as advanced by leading biologist Ludwig von Bertalanffy (1967) and developed by his colleague Paul Weiss (1971) and other members of the interdisciplinary school he founded (Koestler 1978).[4]

In brief, Bertalanffy's general system theory (GST) was conceived "as a unifying research program, as a science of 'wholeness' to overcome or complement mechanistic and reductionist approaches" (Drack and Schwarz 2010). In effect, GST described a research program and a framework rather than a fully fledged body of

[2] Peripheral nervous system.

[3] Central nervous system.

[4] A system was defined by von Bertalanffy (1967) as a set of elements standing in interrelation among themselves and with the environment. GST concerned itself with the scientific exploration of "wholes" and "wholeness" (von Bertalanffy 1967:415). He hoped that the interdisciplinary nature of concepts, models and principles applying to "systems" would provide a possible approach towards the unification of science (von Bertalanffy 1967:415).

theoretical knowledge. Although its aim has not yet been achieved, it is considered to be a signal step towards the science of complexity (Drack and Schwarz 2010; Hofkirchner and Schafranek 2011).

It was therefore premature to apply this as a *model* to explain the vague concept of illness. As a result, Engel's BPS schema is unable to explain how the three dimensions of interest might interact (Quintner et al. 2008). The BPS "model" is best seen as a *conceptual framework*, offering a lens through which to see the clinical world differently, rather than describing how something "works".

Notwithstanding this problem, clinicians working in field of Pain Medicine adopted Engel's approach to illness—as a "model"—to accommodate the psychosocial dimensions of the pain experience, along with its biological dimension (Loeser 1980; Waddell et al. 1984). This adaptation was a major theoretical advance because it reflected the growing recognition of pain as an expression of complex interactions between biological, psychological, social and cultural factors (Gatchel et al. 2007).

Two Nested Conceptual Frameworks

This biopsychosocial framework generated two hierarchical conceptual "models" of the pain experience. The first model was that of Loeser (1980), who proposed four nested domains: nociception, pain, suffering and pain behaviour (Fig. 1).

The Glasgow Illness Model was similarly formulated, with four domains of interest: physical problem, psychological distress, illness behaviour and social interactions (Waddell et al. 1984) (Fig. 2).

Each of these conceptual frameworks includes the moral dimension of "suffering"—explicitly in Loeser's diagram and represented by "psychological distress" in that of Waddell. Importantly, the only observable dimension is the interaction between the person in pain and the surrounding world, described as "pain behaviour" and "illness behaviour" respectively in the two frameworks. In both, the role of the clinician is to determine which dimensions might be determining the person's presentation and to then apply directed therapies.

This exercise requires the clinician not only to be able to differentiate illness behaviour from clinical signs of physical disease but also to detect any mismatch between the amount of demonstrable disease or dysfunction responsible for pain and the level of disability allegedly caused by the pain experience. How these critically important decisions are to be made is left entirely to the discretion of each clinician.

These approaches pose major theoretical and practical problems. Firstly, the frameworks suggest that pain, suffering and behaviour are somehow discrete phenomena, whereas in fact the clinician-observer is unable to make such a distinction. Secondly, although nociception may be understood as a specific physiological process, the other dimensions resist such a reductionist approach. Thirdly, how do the physiological changes of nociception (or other "physical problem") relate

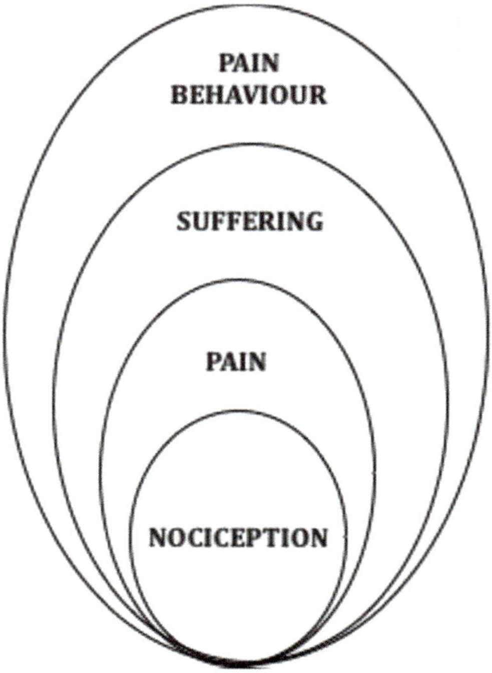

Fig. 1 Loeser's model. From Loeser (1980), with permission

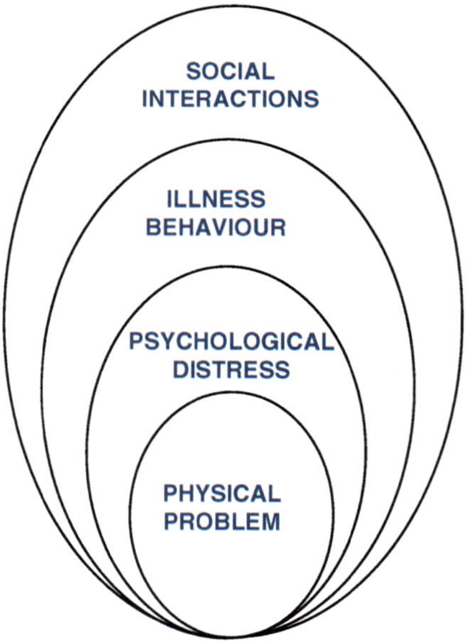

Fig. 2 Glasgow Illness Model. Adapted from Waddell et al. 1984

mechanistically to the other three dimensions? Just as the connection between them is undefinable and arbitrary, so is the pain experience not reducible to neuroscientific explanation (Quintner et al. 2008).

Interestingly, both these frameworks privilege the "objective" view of the clinician when observing the other person's "subjective" pain experience. That is, it is the clinician/observer who decides whether the claimed pain experience is valid. This is despite the stated philosophy of the IASP Task Force that redefined pain (Raja et al. 2020) of privileging the experiencer's perspective. As discussed in chapter "Clarifying the Definition of Pain", that latter stance leads to "pain is what the person says it is", which is unacceptable. In that Chapter, it is argued that an "objective" view should prevail clinically, the responsibility lying with the clinician to determine whether there has been activation of a nociceptive apparatus.

Three Other BPS-Based Explanatory Schemata

A Psychobiological Model

Flor and Hermann (2004) presented an explanatory model based on learning theory. In this view, pain is a multicomponent behavioural response to aversive stimuli. Through prior learning, operant and respondent conditioning, powerful pain memories are formed at all levels of the nervous system. Once established, such pain memories are said to be capable of maintaining pain even in the absence of peripheral nociceptive input.

The individual components (physiological, behavioural-motor and subjective-verbal) of this response are said to reflect the dynamic and continuous interplay between various physiological and psychological factors. However, these same factors are also held to be responsible for the predisposition to and maintenance of chronic pain states, which constitutes the circular reasoning of body–mind dualism.

However, this view takes pain from being a behavioural response (as a symptom) to an experience that may *cause* profound reorganisational changes within the nervous system, thus increasing an individual's susceptibility to all somatosensory input. Here, pain itself is conceptualised as an agent of change—in effect, a "thing".[5] In some way, this emergent aversive response—pain—is capable of changing the very structure of the nervous system, leading to learned memory on the one hand and perpetuating the reorganisational basis of its own genesis on the other. This proposal enshrines a circular argument and accommodates all possibilities, thus constituting a tautology.

---

[5] See chapter "Chronic Pain: A Study in Language and Meaning".

Pain as a Homeostatic Emotion

Influenced by the argument of William James (1884) that emotion is a consequence of bodily change rather than vice versa, Craig suggests that pain is one of many possible human emotions through which the integrity of the body (self) can be maintained in the face of conditions that threaten to disturb its homeostasis (Craig 2003a). In reconceptualising pain as a "homeostatic emotion", he cited then recent neurobiological findings indicating that pain is not part of the exteroceptive somatosensory system but rather "is represented in an unforeseen, novel pathway in humans that is part of a hierarchical system of interoception subserving homeostasis, the sense of the physiological condition of the body (interoception) and the subjective awareness of feelings and emotion" (Craig 2003b).

This pathway of presumed interoception (also termed cenesthesia), which is visible only in primates and well developed only in humans, could be responsible for an individual's subjective awareness of inner body feelings, including emotionality. Craig also proposed that the dorsal margin of the insular cortex contains a primary sensory representation of the activity contained in this pathway (Craig 2002, 2003b).

This claim raises two issues. First, the particular disturbance of homeostasis that gives rise to pain is quite specific, being signalled only through the summated activation of nociceptors, that is, initiated by tissue damage. This is an attempt to unify (old) specificity theory with (new) convergence theory, favouring the former. The second, more profound, issue is that Craig's hypothesis depends on representationism (objectivism) whereby the nervous system is held to mirror an independent world (which includes a "thing" called pain and a sensory image of the physiological condition of the body). Not only is this untestable, but it would require the organism to step outside of itself in order to observe itself, a feat that is not possible.

Pain as a Disease

Another echo of pain as a "thing" in a BPS framework was the attempt to assign disease status to the clinical problem of persistent pain (Siddall and Cousins 2004).[6] It was known that persistent nociception may induce pathoanatomical and pathophysiological changes in the nervous system, including anatomical reorganisation in nociceptive pathways and alterations in patterns of brain activation and cortical topography found in persistent pain states.

These changes were labelled as "secondary pathology" within the nervous system by these authors, who stated that it was "persistent pain [that] does give rise to its own secondary pathology", thus elevating pain to the status of a causative "thing" and constituting a circular argument. They went further by adducing environmental

[6] See chapter "Chronic Pain: A Study in Language and Meaning".

factors as the "tertiary pathology" of pain and thus that pain is "an environmental disease". Such tertiary pathology includes "factors such as genetic makeup, level of spinal inhibition, psychological status and the societal litigation system".

In effect, this proposition was no different from identifying that non-nociceptive factors may be relevant to the pain experience. To label this as "tertiary pathology" was more than a terminological sleight-of-hand, as it carried the implication that these factors can in some unspecified ways contribute to an altered nervous system. But by including "psychological status" as part of this "tertiary pathology", and therefore external to the body, the argument defaulted to the familiar circle of body–mind dualism. Furthermore, what is the pathological basis of the influence, for example, of the "societal litigation system"?

This proposition, of pain-as-a-disease, appears to be concordant with the BPS framework but in fact was a return to the linear causality of the biomedical model.

Sociopsychobiological Frameworks

Critique of BPS "Models"

The proposition of considering different dimensions in the world—somatic, psychological and social—as all contributing to the experience of illness in general and of the pain experience in particular undoubtedly has been a major contribution to broadening the understanding and clinical approach to these phenomena.

However, in the absence of a theory that seeks to understand how the different dimensions interact with each other, these attempts, examples of which were described above, have been caught in circular argument and have been unable to transcend either biomedical reductionism or perpetuation of body-mind dualism. In particular, the implications that pain is a "thing" separate and distinct from the body not only bears little relationship to the lived pain experience but also emphasises the inherent problem that arises when an observer attempts to reduce the "other's" pain experience to predictable parameters (Williamson et al. 2005; Quintner et al. 2008).[7]

This is not to argue against the multi-dimensional approach of BPS frameworks but rather to recognise that thay are not "models" and therefore to recast them as conceptual devices and make them more applicable to the real-world limitations of the clinic.

[7] In fact, the only consistent phenomenon can be nociception, conceptualised as activation of a nociceptive apparatus (See chapter "The Salient Role of Nociception").

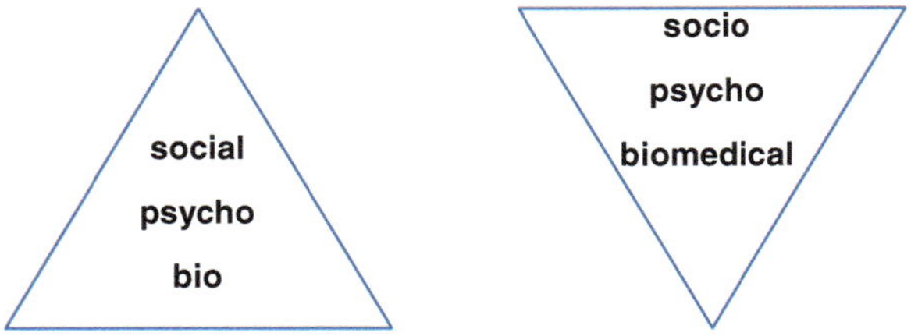

Fig. 3 Inverting the curriculum pyramid. With permission from: Faculty of Pain Medicine, Australian and New Zealand College of Anaesthetists. *Clinical formulation in pain medicine*, 2020

A Sociopsychobiological Framework

Carr and Bradshaw (2014) believed that the current pain curricula, based on BPS, did not provide a coherent viewpoint about pain. Furthermore, standard medical education tended to proceed from a reductionist starting point (featuring anatomical and biochemical studies), then progressing to "higher" levels in the BPS hierarchy.

Believing that a more balanced and holistic conceptualisation of pain was needed for the curriculum, they identified that failure to convey to students the significant contribution of the social dimension to the multidimensional experience of pain meant that the students would not be fully equipped to fulfil their societal obligations to people experiencing pain (Eisenberger 2012).

Because the biomedical dimension of pain (i.e., nociception) is relatively unalterable, Carr and Bradshaw recommended "flipping" the curriculum by giving priority to its sociocultural dimension, namely as "sociopsychobiological" (Fig. 3).

They believed this change in emphasis would enable students to better understand "the intersubjective aspects of a patient's pain, its corrosive effect upon family and other social dynamics, and the relationships between prognosis, disability, and disability payments" (Carr and Bradshaw 2014;13).

A Sociopsychobiomedical Framework

At the same time, in its curriculum revision for training of medical specialists in the discipline of Pain Medicine, the Faculty of Pain Medicine of the Australian and New Zealand College of Anaesthetists adopted the conceptual "inversion" from *biopsychosocial* to *sociopsychobiological*, modifying the latter to *sociopsychobiomedical*, to emphasise its clinical applicability.

To facilitate this application, taking a cue from the Loeser and Waddell diagrams above, this Handbook presents a series of cartoons to capture more coherently the social, psychological and biomedical dimensions of this framework (Fig. 4).

To start at the "biological" or "biomedical" dimension, the (human) organism is conceptualised as a "body" within which is embedded a nervous system and,

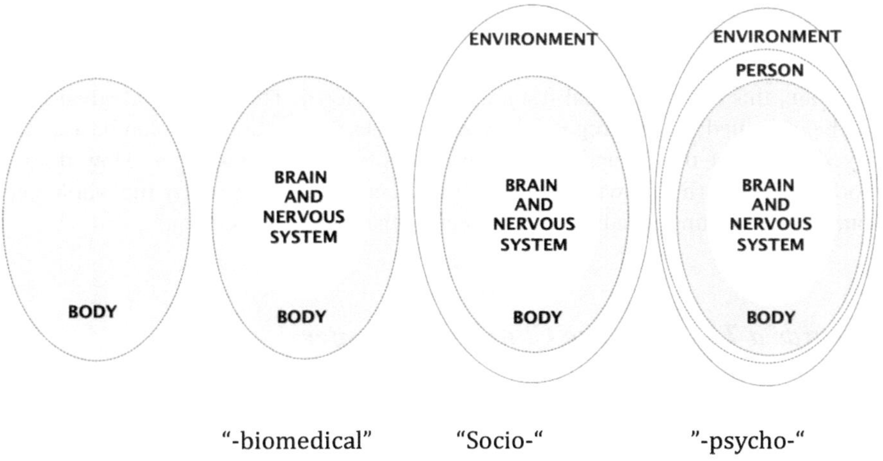

Fig. 4 Building a sociopsychobiomedical framework

Fig. 5 The three dimensions in a sociopsychobiomedical framework

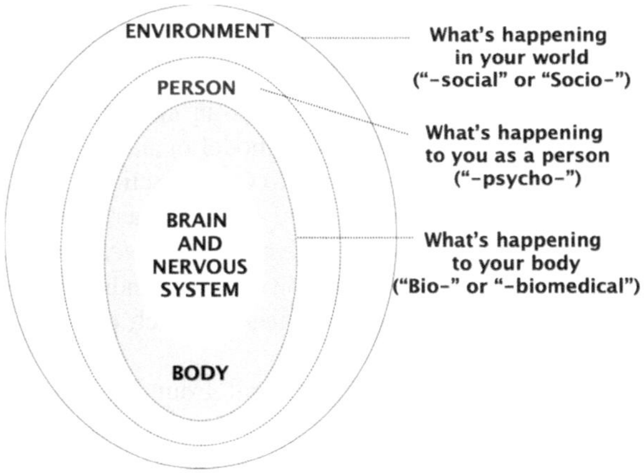

importantly, a brain.[8] This entity exists in an environment with both physical and social features, which constitutes the "social" dimension. Emerging out of the interaction between these two dimensions is what might be characterised as the "person", this constituting the "psychological" dimension.

Figure 5 captures the three dimensions that need to be assessed in the practice of Pain Medicine:

- What is happening in the person's world ("socio-").
- What is happening to the person ("-psycho-").
- What is happening to the person's body ("-biological" or -biomedical") (Fig. 5).

[8] The underlying biology of this dimension is enlarged upon below, under "*Self-referential biological systems*".

The pain experience then may be conceptualised as the interaction—through mechanisms that are largely unknown—of a biological or biomedical dimension, a psychological dimension and a social dimension, as described above.

Again, this is a conceptual framework, not a model. Three potential advantages can be identified: (i) locating the three dimensions as questions that can be asked in any situation of illness or indeed of wellness, without requiring a "How does it work?" answer; (ii) allowing a conceptual space to be occupied by the whole person; and (iii) setting up a basis for dissecting the clinical encounter.[9]

Towards a Theory of the Clinical Encounter

Central to the challenge of trying to understand and thus validate the pain experience is the nature of the clinical encounter itself. This is the pivotal transaction in pain medicine: the presentation by a person distressed because of a perceived threat to their bodily integrity to another person reputed to be learned in the arts and sciences of healing.

The search for a new theoretical perspective to understand this encounter draws on three vantage points (Quintner and Cohen 2016):

(i) the central concept of pain as an *aporia* that cannot be accounted for adequately by the biomedical model or in a biopsychosocial framework, as discussed in chapter "Trying to Gain Traction on a Slippery Subject";
(ii) the nature of humans (and indeed other biological systems) as *autonomous self-organising, self-referential, autopoietic units* that have different perspectives and needs based on the demands of their particular circumstances (which includes the societies in which they are embedded), to be discussed below; and
(iii) *inter-subjectivity* as the natural ground for rapprochement between the world of the clinician and the world of the person experiencing pain, to be discussed in chapter "The Clinical (Two-Person) Encounter".

Broadening the Theory

It has been mentioned that the pain experience is but one way in which an organism signals that a perceived stressor is posing an existential threat (Craig 2003a). Potential "danger" or "stress" stimuli can be physical (tissue damage) or psychological (including environmental), or a combination thereof. Organisms are able to

[9] (iii) will be discussed in chapter "The Clinical (Two-Person) Encounter".

activate evolutionarily conserved stress response systems that are kept under tight control through the mechanism of self-inhibition. According to this hypothesis, chronic pain is but one clinical manifestation of undampened stress response system activation. Other manifestations include fatigue, hyperalgesia, mood disturbance, sleep disturbance and impaired cognition (Lyon et al. 2011).

Self-Organising Biological Systems

Despite General Systems Theory being incomplete (as mentioned above), a critical tenet from it is the capacity of a living organism to change itself in response to perturbations in its environment (Gray 1973; Weiss 1925).

Chilean biologists Humberto Maturana and Francisco Varela (1980) argued that the unique property possessed by living organisms is a particular circular mechanism of spontaneous, autonomous, homeostatic activity contained within a semipermeable boundary, a process that they called autopoiesis, from the Greek, meaning "self-producing".

Autopoiesis refers to the continual production by a system of its own *structure* (its components) and *organisation* (its processes of production). Such a system is said to be self-referential (capable of examining itself) and self-organising (capable of changing and ordering its internal structure according to local rules) and therefore self-sustaining (von Foerster 1960; Luhmann 1995; Luisi 2003).

In order to be autonomous, living systems need to obtain resources from the environment in which they live. Thus, they are at the same time autonomous and dependent (Mariotti 1999). This is a highly negentropic[10] process; that is, one that tends to gain in energy or information, so that input to this complex autopoietic system does not equal its output. From the thermodynamic point of view, such a living system can be said to maintain itself in a state of high statistical improbability of order and organisation: loss of such organisation results in its death.

By contrast the system's structure changes constantly as it continues to adapt itself to disturbances caused by environmental changes. This adaptation of a unity to its environment "is a necessary consequence of that unity's structural coupling with the environment" (Maturana and Varela 1980:102). "Structural coupling" refers to recurrent interactions between two (or more) autopoietic units:

> ... interactions... between unity and environment will consist of reciprocal perurbations. In these interactions, the structure of the environment only *triggers* structural changes in the autopoietic unities (it does not specify or direct them), and vice versa for the environment. The result will be a history of mutual congruent structural changes as long as the autopoetic unity and its containing environment do not disintegrate (Maturana and Varela 1998; 75).

[10] Negentropy is the opposite of entropy, meaning a system is becoming more ordered and structured rather than more disordered or chaotic. It represents the capacity to create and maintain order within a system, often by using energy to counteract the natural tendency toward disorder.

In higher animals, the nervous system, including ultimately the brain, is also an autopoietic unit (Maturana and Varela 1998). In this formulation, the nervous system, including the brain, is not simply a hard-wired computer-like machine that processes only an externally referenced environment, similarly to an incoming telephone line. Rather, it functions like "a hectic family discussion in which a voice (a perturbation) is added to the many voices" and "the consensus of actions reached will not depend on what any particular member of the family says" (Maturana and Varela 1998:163). Another analogy is that of "a group of players engaged in jazz improvisation, and the final result emerges from the continued give and take between them" (Chiel and Beer 1997). These are simple examples of self-organising networks. As such, new patterns or configurations are able to emerge (Varela et al. 1991).

When the person's environment includes another person—another "unity"—such as in the clinical encounter, each triggers changes in the other's structure, and such a reciprocal relationship continues for as long as they remain engaged. During that time, the lived body-environment of each becomes a unique domain of communication (Maturana and Varela 1980).

Importantly, during such interaction, each organism conserves its own autopoiesis and compatibility with its environment. However, the result of that interaction is not determined by a stimulus external to the organism but only by the aggregate state of each organism itself at a given moment (Arbib et al. 1988; Lyon 2004). This is inherently unpredictable.

It is to this domain of communication that chapter "The Clinical (Two-Person) Encounter" turns.

References

Arbib M, Erdi P, Szentagothai J. Structure, function and dynamics: an integrated approach to neural organisation. New York: MIT Press; 1988.

Carr DB, Bradshaw YS. Time to flip the pain curriculum? Anesthesiol. 2014;120:12–4. https://doi.org/10.1097/ALN.0000000000000054.

Chiel HJ, Beer RD. The brain has a body: adaptive behavior emerges from interactions of nervous system, body and environment. Trends Neurosci. 1997;20:553–7. https://doi.org/10.1016/S0166-2236(97)01149-1.

Craig AD. How do you feel? Interoception: the sense of the physiological condition of the body. Nat Rev Neurosci. 2002;8:655–66. https://doi.org/10.1038/nrn894.

Craig AD. A new view of pain as a homeostatic emotion. Trends Neurosci. 2003a;26(6):303–7. https://doi.org/10.1016/S0166-2236(03)00123-1.

Craig AD. Interoception: the sense of the physiological condition of the body. Curr Opin Neurobiol. 2003b;13(4):500–5. https://doi.org/10.1016/s0959-4388(03)00090-4.

Drack M, Schwarz G. Recent developments in general systems theory. Syst Res Behav Sci. 2010;27(6):601–10. https://doi.org/10.1002/sres.1013.

Eisenberger NI. The pain of social disconnection: examining the shared neural underpinnings of physical and social pain. Nat Rev Neurosci. 2012;13:421–34. https://doi.org/10.1038/nrn3231.

Engel GL. The biopsychosocial model and the education of health professionals. Ann N Y Acad Sci. 1978;310:169–81. https://doi.org/10.1016/0163-8343(79)90062-8.

Engel GL. The clinical application of the biopsychosocial model. Am J Psychiatry. 1980;137(5):535–54. https://doi.org/10.1176/ajp.137.5.535.

Flor H, Hermann C. Biopsychosocial models of pain. In: Dworkin RH, Breitbart WS, editors. Psychosocial aspects of pain, progress in pain research and management, vol. 27. Seattle: IASP Press; 2004. p. 47–75.

Follis RH. Cellular pathology and the development of the deficiency disease concept. Bull Hist Med. 1960;34(4):291–317.

Gatchel RJ, Peng YB, Peters ML, Fuchs PN, Turk DC. The biopsychosocial approach to chronic pain: scientific advances and future directions. Psychol Bull. 2007;133(4):581–624. https://doi.org/10.1037/0033-2909.133.4.581.

Gerlee P, Lundh T. Scientific models: red atoms, white lies, and black boxes in a yellow book. Cham: Springer; 2016.

Gray W. Ludwig von Bertalanffy and the development of modern psychiatric thought. In: Gray W, Rizzo ND, editors. Unity through diversity: a festschrift for Ludwig von Bertalanffy, part 1. New York: Gordon and Breach Science Publisher; 1973. p. 169–83.

Hofkirchner W, Schafranek M. General systems theory. In: Hooker C, editor. Philosophy of complex systems. Vol 10 in handbook of the philosophy of science; 2011. p. 177–94. https://doi.org/10.1016/B978-0-444-52076-0.50006-7.

James W. What is an emotion? Mind. 1884;9:188–205.

Koestler A. Janus: a summing up. London: Hutchinson & Co.; 1978.

Loeser JD. Perspectives on pain. In: Turner P, editor. Proceedings of the first world congress on clinical pharmacology and therapeutics. London: Macmillan; 1980. p. 313–6.

Luhmann N. Social systems. Stanford: Stanford University Press; 1995.

Luisi PL. Autopoiesis: a review and a reappraisal. Naturwissenschaften. 2003;90:49–59. https://doi.org/10.1007/s00114-002-0389-9.

Lyon P. Autopoiesis and knowing: reflections on Maturana's biogenic explanation of cognition. Cybern Hum Knowing. 2004;11:21–46.

Lyon P, Cohen ML, Quintner JL. An evolutionary stress-response hypothesis for chronic widespread pain (Fibromyalgia Syndrome). Pain Med. 2011;12:1167–78. https://doi.org/10.1111/j.1526-4637.2011.01168.x.

Mariotti H. Autopoiesis, culture and society. São Paulo: Business School São Paulo; 1999.

Maturana HR, Varela FJ. Autopoiesis and cognition: the realization of the living. Dordrecht: Reidel Publishing Co.; 1980. p. 5–58.

Maturana HR, Varela FJ. The tree of knowledge. The biological roots of human understanding. Paolucci R, translator. Rev. ed. Boston: Shambhala, 1998. 141–176.

McLaren NA. A critical review of the biopsychosocial model. Aust NZ J Psychiatry. 1998;32:86–92. https://doi.org/10.3109/00048679809062712.

Parsons T. The social system. Glencoe: Free Press; 1951.

Quintner J. Why are women with fibromyalgia so stigmatized? Pain Med. 2020;21(5):882–8. https://doi.org/10.1093/pm/pnz350.

Quintner JL, Cohen ML. The challenge of validating the experience of chronic pain: the importance of intersubjectivity and reframing. In: Van Rysewyck S, editor. Meanings of pain. Cham: Springer; 2016. p. 281–93.

Quintner JL, Buchanan D, Cohen ML, Katz JD, Williamson OD. Pain medicine and its models: helping or hindering? Pain Med. 2008;9:824–34. https://doi.org/10.1111/j.1526-4637.2007.00391.x.

Radden J. The philosophy of mind and psychiatry. Curr Opin Psychiatry. 1999;12:589–92.

Raja SN, Carr DB, Cohen M, et al. The revised IASP definition of pain: concepts, challenges, and compromise. Pain. 2020;161(9):1976–82. https://doi.org/10.1097/j.pain.0000000000001939.

Reber AS. The penguin dictionary of psychology. Harmondsworth: Penguin Books Ltd.; 1985. p. 738–9.

Siddall PJ, Cousins MJ. Persistent pain as a disease entity: implications for clinical management. Anesth Analg. 2004;99:510–20.

Varela FJ, Thompson E, Rosch E. The embodied mind. Cambridge, MA: The MIT Press; 1991. p. 87–103.

von Bertalanffy L. The model of open systems: beyond molecular biology. In: Breck AD, Yourgran W, editors. Biology, history and natural philosophy. New York: Plenum Press; 1967. p. 17–30.

von Foerster H. On self-organizing systems and their environments. In: Yovits M, Cameron S, editors. Self-organizing systems. London: Pergamon Press; 1960. p. 31–50.

Waddell G, Bircher M, Finlayson D, Main CJ. Symptoms and signs: physical disease or illness? Br Med J. 1984;289:739–41. https://doi.org/10.1136/bmj.289.6447.739.

Wade DT, Halligan PW. Do biomedical models of illness make for good healthcare systems? Br Med J. 2004;329:1398–401. https://doi.org/10.1136/bmj.329.7479.1398.

Weiss PA. Tierisches Verhalten als 'Systemreaktion'. Die Orienterung der Ruhstellungen von Schmetterlingen (Vanessa) gegen Licht und Schwerkraft. Biol Gen. 1925;1:165–248.

Weiss PA. The basic concept of hierarchic systems. In: Weiss P, editor. Hierarchical organized systems in theory and practice. New York: Hafner; 1971. p. 1–43.

Williamson OD, Buchanan DA, Quintner JL, Cohen ML. Pain beyond monism and dualism [letter]. Pain. 2005;116:169–70. https://doi.org/10.1016/j.pain.2005.04.011.

The Clinical (Two-Person) Encounter

Abstract The clinical "two-person" encounter between the clinician and the person experiencing pain is characterised by complexity, uncertainty and unpredictability. This chapter seeks to understand why what should be a basic function of health professionals—the clinical management of people experiencing persistent pain—is not only unsatisfactory in terms of therapeutic outcomes, but also frustrating for both patient and clinician, each of whom is seeking validation from the other.

A number of similar but sufficiently different conceptual frameworks for how the clinical "game" is actually played is presented. The central concept in all of these is that of *intersubjectivity*, as coined by Edmund Husserl (1859–1938), which essentially implies a willingness to see the world from the other's point of view and to appreciate how the other person makes sense of their being in the shared world. A parallel framework is offered by Pierre Bourdieu (1930–2002). These approaches are compared with others, to offer clinicians pathways to more easily navigate this fundamental process in pain medicine.

The potential is explored for using these approaches to achieve validation of both predicaments—that of the person experiencing pain and that of the clinician seeking to assist. This may lead to some innovative approaches and strategies towards more satisfactory ethical and therapeutic outcomes for both parties.

When Engel's biopsychosocial (BPS) model of illness was adapted for use in the context of clinical pain, as discussed in chapter "Conceptual Frameworks", the interpersonal or "two-person" hierarchical level was not addressed. This chapter describes a number of ways in which BPS-based frameworks might be operationalised at this level. Central to this exercise is the concept of intersubjectivity, as it might relate both to the individual experiencing pain and to the clinician providing care in that situation. An exploration of the dynamics of the clinical encounter will show possibilities for both parties to achieve mutual validation of their respective predicaments.

M. Cohen, J. Quintner, *A Philosophical Handbook for Pain Medicine Practice*,
https://doi.org/10.1007/978-981-92-1682-6_6

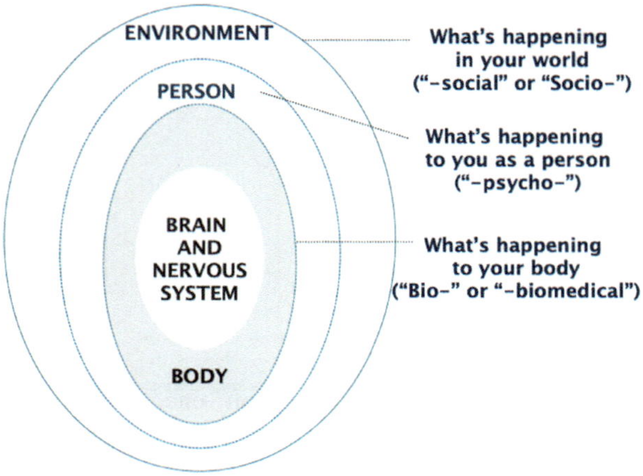

Fig. 1 A sociopsychobiomedical framework

In chapter "Conceptual Frameworks", a conceptual diagram of the sociopsychobiomedical framework (Fig. 1) for thinking about pain was introduced:

In the clinical encounter, there are two people (autopoietic units) interacting in the same social environment (structural coupling). This environment might be called the "biopsychosocial space"; it has also been termed the "intersubjective space" (Husserl 1973) and the "third space" (Winnicott 1971). In this space, the lived body-environment of each becomes a unitary structure that emerges through their reciprocal interaction (Maturana and Varela 1987). Importantly, each organism conserves its own autopoiesis and compatibility with its environment (Varela et al. 1991). From a patient's report of a pain experience to a clinician, it can already be inferred that an important change has occurred in that person's nervous system following an exposure to a particular perturbation and that their efforts to adapt to it have been unsuccessful (Fig. 2).

Intersubjectivity: Insights from Husserl's Philosophy

In simple terms, intersubjectivity refers to "the process and product of sharing experiences, knowledge, understandings and expectations with others".[1] The most comprehensive treatise on intersubjectivity is the work of the philosopher Edmund Husserl who coined the term. His writings on the topic extend over 50 years, and cover a very wide range of meanings and phenomena (Duranti 2010).

One thesis of this chapter is that Husserl's template for exploring inter-subjectivity can be a basis for understanding the two-person encounter in the pain clinic. As will be shown, his template meshes with the insights of many others who have contributed to this understanding.

[1] Oxford reference.com; accessed 09 Aug 24.

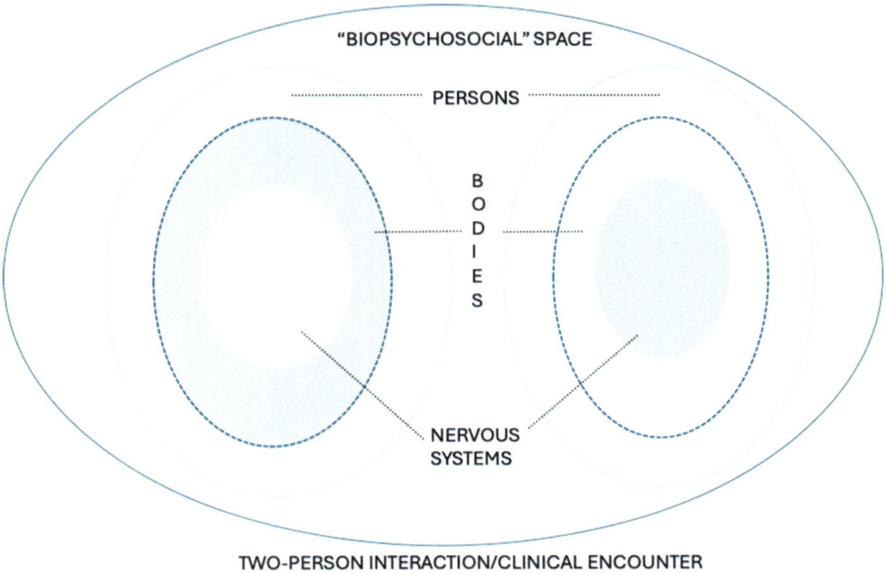

Fig. 2 Conceptualising the two-person encounter in a sociopsychobiomedical framework

For Husserl, intersubjectivity denotes the possibility of being in the same place as or even exchanging places with the other person, which implies a willingness to see the world from the other's point of view and to appreciate how the other person makes sense of their being in the shared world (Husserl 1973).

Husserl (1973) described four domains of intersubjective interaction:

(i) Being-apart-from-one-another (*Auseinandersein*)
(ii) Being-with-one-another (*Miteinandersein*)
(iii) Being-within-one-another (*Ineinandersein*)
(iv) Being-for-one-another (*Füreinandersein*)

Being-Apart-From-One-Another (Auseinandersein)

Husserl conceptualised humans as singular autonomous subjects (*monads*), living apart in a community of other similarly singular subjects, each performing different social roles (Strasser 1975). By referring to them as *monads*, he not only reflected the ontological stance of the philosopher Gottfried Leibniz but also anticipated modern biological understandings of autonomy (Varela 2025).

Both these philosophers were concerned with the ultimate constituents of the universe to which the entire created world is reducible (Glover 2008). Leibniz' claim was that "the universe ultimately consists of indivisible, immaterial

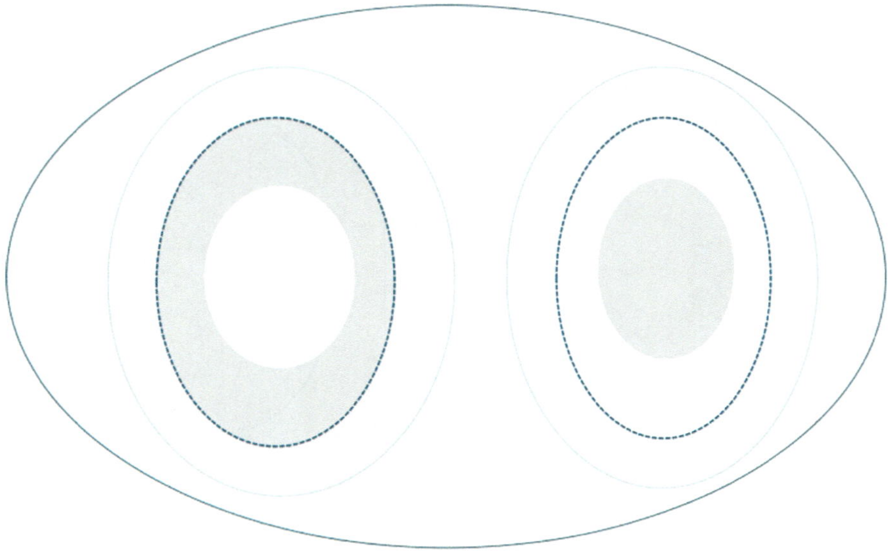

Fig. 3 Conceptualising "being apart from one another" in the two-person encounter

substances – *monads* – that do not causally interact with each other …" (Strickland 2020:209). This meant that *monad*s are quite independent with respect to one another. Each *monad* contains a unique script or program of divine origin that Leibniz described as "an internal principle of change".

Husserl's views of monadism aligned with those of Leibniz. But in stark contrast, Husserl focussed on the conscious self that must underlie all human thought and perception. In his ontology, "every consciousness is singular, non-repeatable, individual; it is absolutely independent of every other consciousness" (Strasser 1975:3). The key assertion is that although monads are considered to be self-sufficient at any given moment in time, they must interact with others in the community, whether by choice or by necessity, to ensure their survival.

Maturana and Varela's biological ontology of living beings bears a striking convergence with the monadic philosophical ontology of Husserl (Maturana and Varela 1980). In both ontologies, individuals are portrayed as pre-programmed to be autonomous and separate from their surroundings but nonetheless dependent upon them for continued survival.

Husserl's domain of *Auseinandersein* can therefore be reconceptualised in the two-person encounter as recognition of, and respect for, each individual's fundamental biological **autonomy**.

This is captured diagrammatically as shown above (Fig. 3).

Being-With-One-Another (Miteinandersein)

Husserl introduced the notion of a multi-layered and complex *life-world*, built upon tradition, incorporating "the sedimented achievements of generations of anonymous others" (Moran 2017:112). He used the analogy of a flowing stream of experiences for the repository of such achievements, one of which is language. The same repository contains other shared values, shared habits, traditions, rituals, collective memories and even collective emotions, all of which serve to bind communities together (Szanto 2015).

These considerable achievements need to be acknowledged and factored into engagements between humans because they can "affect, modulate or even bias not only intergroup, but also interpersonal understanding" (Szanto 2015:448). In other words, we share a common world in which we act and suffer together (Moran 2012). A particular instance of this phenomenon is pain, which can be seen as a mutually recognised if not necessarily shared experience (Cohen et al. 2018).

Husserl's *Miteinandersein* domain can be reconceptualised in the two-person clinical encounter as recognition of and respect for the essential *humanity* shared by both parties, and can be captured diagrammatically as shown below (Fig. 4):

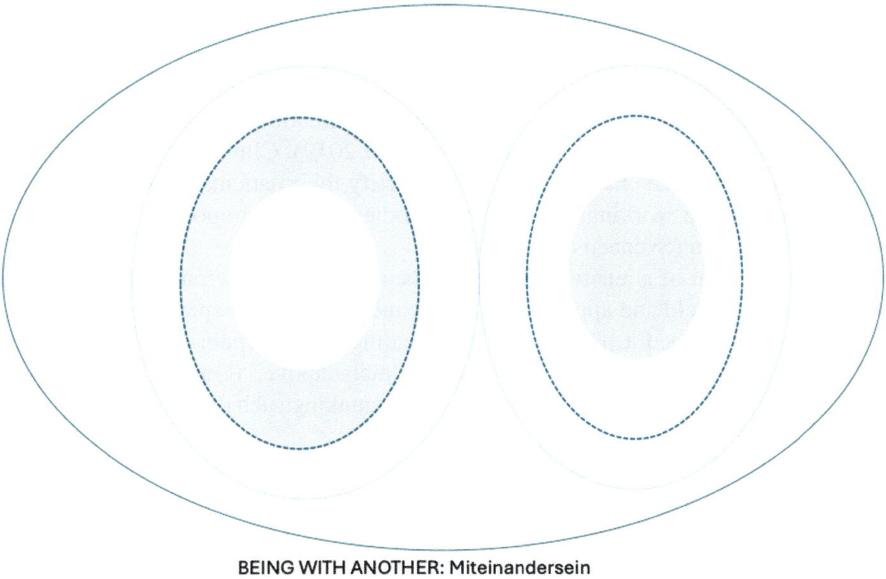

Fig. 4 Conceptualising "being with one another" in the two-person encounter

Being-Within-One-Another (Ineinandersein)

Husserl (1973) argued that communal life of separate individuals would not be possible if we were not able, to some extent, to anticipate the wishes, intentions, worries, doubts and hopes of others. This incorporation of the other person into one's inner life can be achieved by reflecting about them, utilising available knowledge of the person and their background, as well as drawing upon one's memory and imagination. This process underlies the concept of empathy which, for Husserl, arises out of "our exposure to their bodies moving and acting in ways we recognise as similar to the ways we would act in similar circumstances" (Duranti 2010:8).

Edith Stein, Husserl's pupil, understood empathy as "a way of knowing what the other person is experiencing", rather than being an emotional response to that knowledge (Meneses and Larkin 2012:158). For Stein (1917/1989), empathy is "neither contagion, nor imitation, nor sympathy", nor is it "any form of intellectually reasoned knowledge about another's experience" (Meneses and Larkin 2012:164). Her views accord with those of Scheler (1954), who, like Husserl, believed that we automatically gain access to the experienced life of others through their expressive phenomena such as laughter, tears, blushing, gnashing of teeth, tenor of speech and fist clenching.

As expounded by Husserl, Stein and Scheler, empathy is mediated through our learned understanding of the signs, sounds, movements and gestures of others (Owen 2000). It is through awareness of the body of the other person that the clinician can observe behaviours that indicate patients' distress, including the pain experience.

Clinicians who use their own pain experience as an indication of how their patients might be feeling when facing a similar situation must not presume that these two perspectives will coincide (Overgaard 2019). Clinicians also need to be aware that their "gaze" has the power to objectify their patients, making them feel alienated from the workings of their own bodies, thereby imposing an additional burden upon them (Svenaeus 2009:121).

A similar form of alienation can arise when the clinician wrongly interprets the negative beliefs held and appraisals made by individual pain experiencers. Here the clinician has assumed a judicial role by deciding whether pain-related cognitions and behaviour of patients are "adaptive" or "maladaptive" (Quintner et al. 2011). The points of reference used by clinicians when making such decisions would seem to be quite arbitrary.

Finally, as "Scheler and others have recognised … Empathy may not be benign or caring for others" (Moran 2022:27). Such examples include pretending, lying, deceiving, spin-doctoring, acting, emotionally manipulating or influencing the other person (Moran 2022).

Husserl's *Miteinandersein* domain can be reconceptualised in the two-person encounter as the practice of *empathy* (Fig. 5):

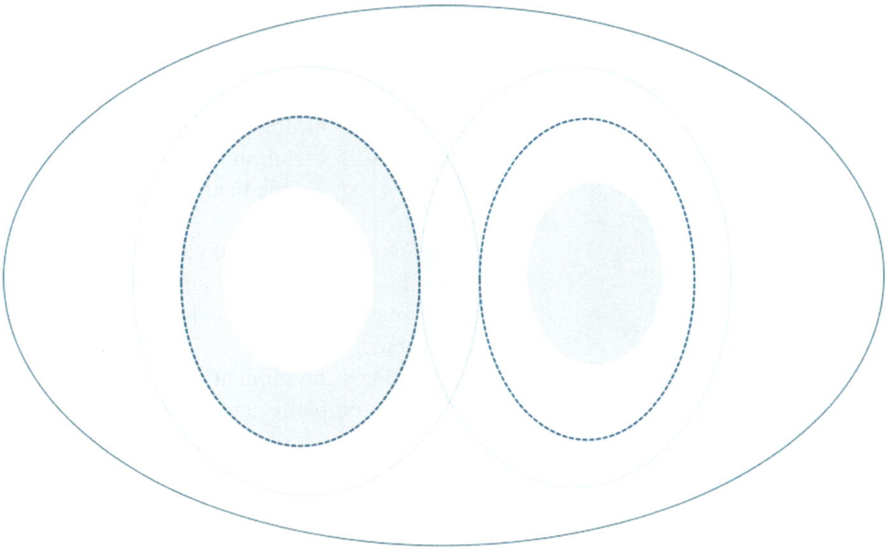

Fig. 5 Conceptualising "being within one another" in the two-person encounter

Being-for-One-Another (Füreinandersein)

Husserl assigned primacy to the ego (the conscious self) within an intersubjective relationship. In his Fifth Cartesian Meditation (1960), he warned that the other person might be a target for "projection of passive non-conscious processes, whereby my experiences become given as belonging to the other" (Quoted by Owen 2000:7). People seeking help are vulnerable and susceptible to attempts at manipulation and control (Calnan and Rowe 2008).

Nonetheless, it is self-evident that "being-for-one-another" implies that each party to an intersubjective engagement will come to trust the other. In everyday life, trust, concisely defined as the belief that someone is honest and reliable, is a very fluid and varied entity, being contingent and context dependent. It is best seen as "a relational quality that emerges from the interaction" (Cohn 2015:5). Furthermore, "it cannot be rigorously demarcated from other associated qualities – such as mistrust and distrust" (Cohn 2015:7). Even so, in an empathetic clinical encounter, clinician and patient each take a step further to carve out a common space of signs and understandings based on trust (Favareau 2002).

The ethical responsibility imposed upon the clinician working in this common space is to show compassion, as expressed by Pullman (2002:85) in the context of pain medicine practice:

> Although we cannot feel another's pain, the shared meanings occasioned by intersubjective consciousness enable us to suffer along with one another.

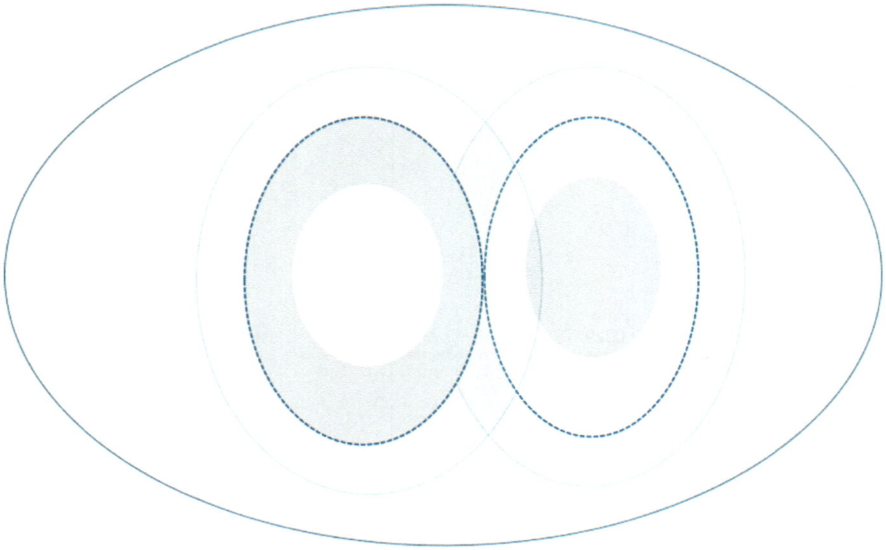

Fig. 6 Conceptualising "being for one another" in the two-person encounter

It is also the clinician's responsibility to try to transcend their own implicit bias in order to reach an understanding of the patient, unclouded by personal assumptions and judgements. However, some clinicians may selflessly give too much of themselves, believing that they have done so for the greater good and with the hope that it will be appreciated by their patient. Although this form of giving might make them feel good about themselves, it also makes them more prone to burnout, depression and suicide (Blum 2019). Matthias et al. (2010) showed that caregivers who are unable to relieve their patient's pain can feel frustrated, ungratified and even guilty.

In summary, each party can bring elements of pre-understanding, fore-meanings, prejudice, openness to change, idiosyncratic language, mythology and imaginative scenarios to the engagement:

> … the doctor's encounter with the patient can enable them to see new horizons. We cannot simply drop in a story or horizon. We need to help them to a new understanding and always remember that the patient's horizon and ours are different. (Clark 2008:58)

Husserl's *Füreinandersein* domain can be reconceptualised in the two-person encounter as the establishment and maintenance of *trust* (Fig. 6):

To summarise, the four domains of intersubjectivity, as explored by Husserl, that might characterise the two-person encounter are respect for the other's autonomy, recognition of shared humanity, empathy but not emotional contagion and establishment of trust. Although the series of cartoons might suggest an axis of increasing intimacy, these domains are not discrete and not exclusive; they are better seen as concurrent rather than as progressive stages of engagement. The degree to which one or more domain might be predominant at any time can neither be prescribed nor known beforehand. Each clinical encounter is therefore a unique event for each party and much negotiation may be needed before a state of mutually acceptable stability in the relationship is attained.

Insights from Bourdieu's Sociology

Another approach to examining the dynamics of this two-person interaction can be taken from the writings of the French philosopher and sociologist Pierre Bourdieu (Collyer et al. 2015), as applied to clinical medicine by Frank (2002) and to medical education by Gomes and Rego (2013). This framework, which can be seen as either complementary or alternative to a sociopsychobiomedical approach, turns on Bourdieu's concepts of *illusio*, *habitus*, *field* and *capital*.

Similarly to Husserl, Bourdieu's starting point within an intersubjective relationship is the conscious self.

Illusio

Bourdieu and Wacquant (1992) coined the term *illusio*,[2] to describe the kinds of discourse in which a person can take part as a player in their own and in other people's social games. In such games, Bourdieu argues, *all* actions by individuals are interest-driven, regardless of the context in which they are undertaken. Self-interest is the driving force of human behaviour, as individuals try to maximise their gains and accumulate resources under different forms of capital (economic, social, cultural, symbolic; see below) (Navarro 2006:14). This is the main determinant of social arrangements in any specific field.

The clinical encounter can be viewed as one such social game, which both parties are strongly encouraged to take seriously as the stakes can be high (Frank 2002). The essence of a clinical encounter is dialogue, captured by Frank (2002) as "talk grounded in mutual desire to recognise and be recognised".

Although in practice they can overlap, three standard forms of discourse—or "game" in this encounter—can be identified:

- the objective discourse of factuality, informed by science, as the basis of biomedical practice;
- the subjective discourse, the realm of personal expressiveness (although its importance tends to be diminished in the medical context); and
- the intersubjective or social discourse, emphasising negotiation towards shared meaning.

To each of these forms of *illusio*, the players bring their own *habitus* and *field*.

[2] Derived from the Latin root "lus-" related to "ludere" meaning "to play" or "to game".

Habitus

The *habitus* of an individual is the set of embodied habits, tastes, actions, styles and attitudes that are acquired through the process of growing up in families, communities and societies (Bourdieu 1994). This constitutes a primer for how people think and act in accordance with a particular social context.

People's experiences become embodied in their *habitus*, and through them they develop a "feel for the game", learning the rules that eventually become second nature to them (Bourdieu 1994). Moreover, "these habits are not just individual ways of behaving, but include lasting decisions, values and judgments made by an individual that have been adopted in the course of his or her life" (Moran 2011).

In practical terms, *habitus* embodies "know-how" in managing day-to-day life situations, and is a predictive model of behaviours in response to specific circumstances that call for action (Gomes and Rego 2013). In this context of medical education, *habitus* "… is not the simple internalisation of social rules, rather it is a dynamic interaction between individuals, social agents and social structure in order to enable acting-in-the-world" (hyphens added) (Gomes and Rego 2013).

Applied to medical practice, *habitus* conditions clinicians' ways of "being, seeing, acting and thinking" (Emmerich 2013). It follows that clinician and patient each brings to the clinical encounter not only their own *habitus* but also the "mutual desire to recognise and be recognised" (Frank 2002).

Field

The encounter takes place in what Bourdieu (1975) termed a *field*, a structured space in which agents and their respective social positions are located. The field determines the limits or boundaries of the space in which *habitus* operates.

The field is an arena of struggle for "possession of goods, services, knowledge, or status and the competition among agents to monopolise distinct capitals" (Navarro 2006:18). It can be looked at as "a big game where the participating agents, owners and knowers of the rules dispute positions of specific dominance and profits" (Gomes and Rego 2013:262). The position of each particular agent in the *field* is a result of dynamic interactions between the specific rules of the *field*, the agent's *habitus* and what Bourdieu termed the agent's *capital*, that refers to the kinds of resources agents bring to the social interaction or the products of those interactions.

Capital

The concept of *capital* is the third component of the *illusio*, along with *habitus* and *field* (Bourdieu 1986). This concept includes all forms of valued resources, comprising economic capital (concerned with material resources), social capital

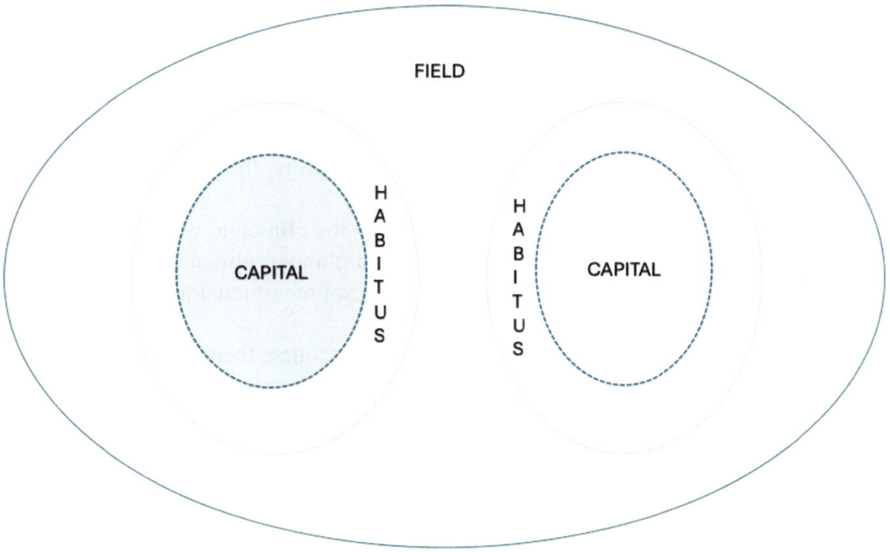

Fig. 7 Conceptualising the two-person encounter using Bourdieu's terms

(an enduring network of mutual acquaintances), cultural capital (the cultural competencies individuals develop through socialisation and learn over time) and symbolic capital (which is anchored in culture to ensure interaction and communication, but also to create and maintain social hierarchies) (Navarro 2006:15).

For contemporary health care professionals, prestige, reputation and fame have become valued forms of symbolic capital, which can be incorporated as skills and knowledge, objectivised in books or tools or institutionalised as degrees or certificates (Abel and Frohlich 2012).

The diagrammatic schema employed above can be applied to Bourdieu's *illusio* in the context of the two-person encounter (Fig. 7):

Application of Bourdieu's Concepts to Medicine

In Western medical practice, the rules of the game are well understood, if infrequently articulated. Society expects clinicians to be trained primarily to apply basic scientific principles of diagnosis and treatment to the injured or diseased human body in order to return it to functional health.

In relation to medical education, Gomes and Rego (2013) draw on Bourdieu's concepts:

> Considering medicine as a socially structured space where social agents, namely physicians and those who intend to gain this title - medical students—meet and follow rules and principles of regulation specific to that occupation, it would appear that this profession can function … as a well-organised model for Bourdieu's field.

Bourdieu saw the locus of these interactions in the scientific field as being "a competitive struggle in which the specific issue at stake is the monopoly of scientific authority or … the monopoly of scientific competence in the sense of a particular agent's socially recognised capacity to speak and act legitimately (i.e. in an authorised and authoritative way) in scientific matters" (Bourdieu 1975:19). Substitute "clinical" for "scientific", and these comments capture the *field* of the clinical encounter.

The patient is expected to present symptoms to the clinician, who then evaluates them in order to arrive at a specific diagnosis and plan a regimen of treatment. But when these societal expectations cannot be met, a source of tension becomes apparent in the clinical encounter.

A struggle for dominance in this field-specific discourse then ensues between the agents over whose interpretation of the patient's predicament in the world should prevail. A possibly challenging example of this was encountered in chapter "Clarifying the Definition of Pain", where it was proposed that the perspective of the clinician-observer should prevail over that of the pain experiencer in terms of determining whether that reported experience is concordant with the definition of pain. Other examples of such contested interpretations include the notion of pain functioning as a bodily protector and Pain Reprocessing Therapy, both of which are dissected in chapter "Errors in Language and Logic Call for Epistemic Discipline".

The use of language by medical practitioners provides clues as to how they might bring their *habitus* as a form of benevolent possessor of their patients to the *field* (Horton 2003). Even the use of the word "patient" implying someone waiting for something to be done to alleviate their suffering, and the way in which patients become "subjects" in research studies, exemplify these unconsciously adopted paternalistic attitudes that can strip sick people of their unique characteristics.

The historical outcome of health professionals' persistent search for accumulation of *capital* is "to entrench hierarchies that in turn require permanent vigilance to legitimise and maintain these social differences, or a continuous effort to keep 'misrecognition' of the origins of these asymmetries" (Navarro 2006:14).

When such social capital becomes legitimised as part of a dominant culture, Bourdieu's concept of *symbolic violence* can come into play (Bourdieu 1990). Pringle (1998) explains how this concept relates to her particular medical specialty:

> His account applies well to the field of internal medicine where, it may be argued, power and prestige are maintained through forms of symbolic violence, 'gentle, invisible … unrecognised as such, chosen, as much as undergone, that of trust, obligation, personal loyalty, hospitality, gifts, debts, piety, in a word, of all the virtues honoured by the ethics of honour.

Horton (2003) also sees the unstated terms and conditions of the doctor-patient relationship as one that may be more appropriate as being between master and servant. Typical examples of "medical master" discourses in chronic pain include:

- the biomedical narrative, reducing the patient to a mere organism in the hands of a techno-scientific apparatus;

- the bio-behavioural story where, for example, a person's pain is seen as a conditioned response;
- the egotistic clinician narrative, where social standing and career goals overshadow patient needs;
- the ironic-sarcastic discourse, which though superficially friendly, barely conceals the clinician's contempt for the patient's preferred explanatory story; and
- above all others, the stigmatising narrative by which the patient is declared an immoral *malade imaginaire.*[3]

The "medical master" discourse reflects tension between the social or symbolic capital of the health care professional and that of the patient-person experiencing chronic pain. It may explain how clinicians' inability to relieve pain might threaten their own social capital.

An important aspect of social capital for people experiencing pain is their access to reliable and up-to-date scientific information and therefore to clear assessment and treatment pathways, which is the province of health care professionals (Nielsen 2012). When such information is not conveyed appropriately and accurately, the patient's social capital is threatened and trust in that health care professional will be undermined. When it comes to the needs of people experiencing pain, all such master-servant narratives may be seen as unethical options for medical practice.

Parallels Between BPS and Bourdieu Approaches

Diagrammatically, Bourdieu's and BPS approaches can be compared (Fig. 8):

Here, the *body* (with its embedded nervous system) is shown to correspond with *capital*, both being characterised by relative immutability, while *person* and *habitus* also tend to correspond and, although characterised by their established nature, may be more amenable to change. However, perhaps it is the arena of the third set of correspondences, in the structured space of *environment* or *field*, where there is the most potential for resolution of tension and therefore for enhancing the effectiveness of the clinical encounter.

Other Approaches to the Two-Person Encounter

Some perspectives on reconstituting the *environment* or *field* of the clinical encounter come from an examination of the roles of intersubjectivity and the "third space" through empathy and social prospection (Crisp 2015).

[3] See Molière's "The Imaginary Invalid".

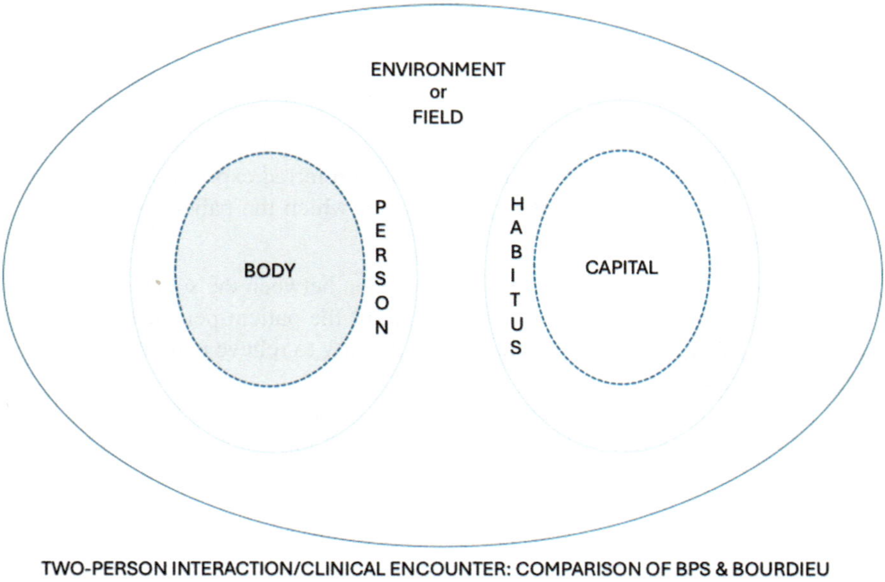

Fig. 8 Comparing biopsychosocial and Bourdieu conceptions of the two-person encounter

The Intersubjective ("Third") Space: Buber and Winnicott

In his most influential work, the philosopher Martin Buber (1878–1965) outlined two different approaches through which people can choose to relate to others: that of *I-It* or *I-Thou* (Buber 1937).

The biomedical model of illness has traditionally employed the *I-It* approach or paternalistic model (Charles et al. 1997), where the patient is portrayed as a passive recipient of treatment, with which cooperation is expected.

By contrast, echoing Buber's *I-Thou* approach, intersubjectivity refers to one's ability to interact with others in a reciprocal and mutually meaningful fashion (Grinnell 1983). They live in what Buber calls "the between", the relational space created by the encounter.

In a similar vein, the realisation of intersubjectivity takes place within the "third space", as conceptualised by paediatrician and psychoanalyst Donald Winnicott (1896–1971). Bearing a resemblance to the imaginative play of children, the "third space" can be likened to that in which the players are able construct a relevant culture for a particular purpose (Winnicott 1971).

In relation to the clinical encounter, clinician and patient seek to carve out a shared space of signs and understandings created by their respective actions (Favareau 2002). In effect, this space constitutes a *field* of Bourdieu where the *habitus* of each player is respected (Emmerich 2013).

This form of clinician-patient interaction is also an example of Frank's "ethics-in-process", taking place in a virtual space that both parties have agreed to enter for the purpose of creating a therapeutic relationship (Frank 2004). It functions as an "in-between" or transitional space between subject and object (Praglin 2006) where a truly ethical culture of clinical practice can be developed and each can live in the other's experience. This space can then become a zone of active exchange, where dynamic negotiation and testing of boundaries are allowed to take place.

The intersubjective space is "where one finds the most authentic and creative aspects of our personal and communal existence, including artistic, scientific, and religious expression" (Praglin 2006). Through creative expression, situations can be resolved and new possibilities are allowed to emerge. Thus, the clinician-patient relationship becomes a truly intersubjective one, when Buber's *I-Thou* dichotomy can be unified as "*We*".

Social Prospection

In his important "contact hypothesis", Allport (1954) suggested that bringing together members of different groups under appropriate conditions could lead to more positive inter-group relations.

Crisp and Turner (2012) expanded Allport's hypothesis to encompass "the planning, rehearsal, and enacting interactions with others – the ability to mentally time-travel that is necessary to transcend people's tendencies to see out-groups as 'them', and to see a possible future in which they are also 'us'". They assembled evidence in support of the proposition that by simply imagining contact with a member of an "out" group a person is engaging in conscious processes that parallel those involved in actual contact.

Crisp and colleagues (Crisp and Turner 2012; Miles and Crisp 2014; Crisp 2015) developed this theme as *social prospection*, defined as "the capacity to mentally project oneself into the past or the future to consider alternative perspectives based on our past experiences". This would appear to run parallel with empathy.

The potential benefits of a person imagining a positive interaction with an out-group member include positive changes in attitudes and behaviour towards the member, as well as less overall anxiety for the person involved. In addition, they draw on research from other areas of behavioural science that shows that social prospection can enhance self-efficacy.

Evidence assembled by Miles and Crisp (2014) also supports the proposition that imagined contact is potentially a key component of educational strategies aiming to promote positive social change. Although this has not been tested in relation to clinicians and their patients experiencing pain, it has been shown on the one hand that only providing information does not change intergroup attitudes. On the other hand, imagined contact could help to challenge existing attitudes and to "reduce anxiety and negative expectations about contact, while generating positive emotions like empathy" (Crisp and Turner 2012).

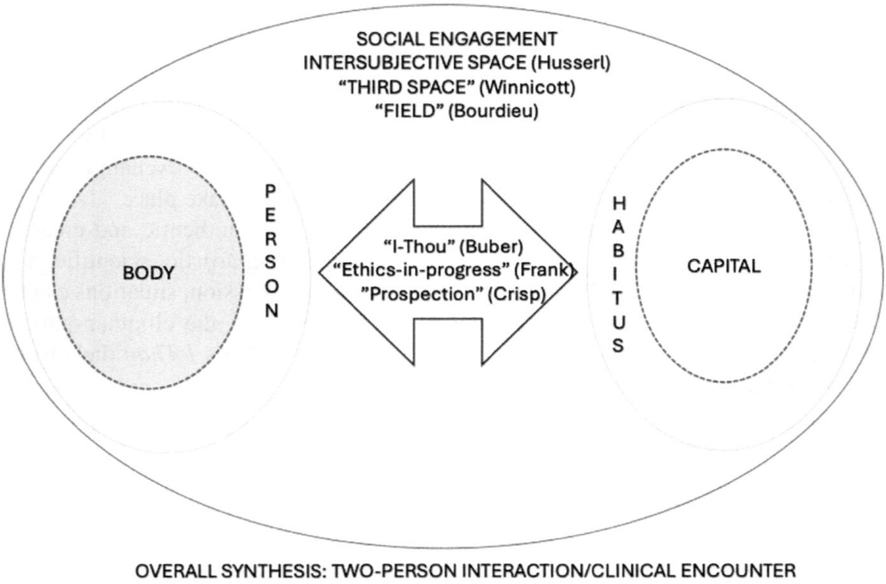

Fig. 9 Overview of the two-person encounter

Social prospection may be a novel template for reframing the clinical encounter in pain medicine.

These other approaches also can be captured in the same diagrammatic schema (Fig. 9):

Using the Two-Person Encounter to Negotiate Towards Validation

Reframing the Concept of Validation

Validation was defined in chapter "Conceptual Frameworks" as meaning confirmation, corroboration or substantiation. When applied to the person experiencing chronic pain, there are two aspects of this process. The first is the recognition and affirmation by the clinician of where-they-are-in-the-world and the second is a mutually agreed reframing of the person's predicament.

Drawing upon an older connotation of the word "validation", namely to "strengthen", can add a third, ethical aspect to the role of the physician.

Through the act of "being with" the patient-experiencing-pain in the intersubjective space (*Miteinandersein*, or respect for shared humanity) and negotiating an interpretation of the patient's narrative through dialogical discourse, the clinician may be able to provide a satisfactory explanation of the patient's predicament and lay the groundwork for the patient to play an active role in addressing it. The strength of this approach is that it increases the likelihood of adherence to prescribed therapy, and implementation of strategies of self-monitoring, self-management and self-efficacy.

However, such an approach may be resisted by agents of the dominant ideology, whose "task of teaching medicine leans towards cultural and social reproduction … that, in effect intends to perpetuate the existing *symbolic capital*" (Gomes and Rego 2013).

Reframing the Problem Through Narrative

Child psychologist Colwyn Trevarthen (1979) suggested that in humans, the pain experience is fundamentally associated with the need to tell someone about it. For those experiencing chronic pain, where there may be no readily discernible lesion or process, being in the intersubjective space provides a unique opportunity for them to tell their story to their clinician and for both to use the process of dialogical discourse to reframe the problem.

In contrast to monologic discourse, which pretends to be the ultimate word, finalised and deaf to the other's response, dialogic discourse is the willingness to become caught up in the other's *illusio*, at least provisionally (Frank 2002). From a dialogical standpoint, listening is the capacity to share what makes someone's story worth telling and worth hearing. The dialogical and profoundly ethical task is for each to see themselves as participants in the other's story to the extent that "each feels implicated in the other's life story, and feels that other's implication in his or her own story - and believes these stories matter, crucially" (Frank 2002).

The traditional medical narrative, which is based upon the discovery of an underlying disease process, cannot be the only one available for the person experiencing chronic pain. To meaningfully engage with their patients at a deeper level, clinicians need to offer a continuous narrative that might lead the patient to an existential understanding of their predicament. One such reframing narrative is to make both parties aware that humans share fundamental biological properties in common with all living organisms, and that the pain experience can often be associated with many clinical features suggesting that activation of evolutionarily conserved systems of stress or sickness response has occurred (Lyon et al. 2011).

This biological narrative transcends dualistic thinking, as the clinical problem can be reframed as one due to dysregulation of the mechanisms that control or regulate these processes. Invoking a system such as the organism's nociceptive apparatus (Cohen et al. 2023) that may well be activated by both physical stressors through "upward" causative mechanisms and psychological and social stressors through "downward" causative mechanism is one example.

References

Abel T, Frohlich KL. Capitals and capabilities: linking structure and agency to reduce health inequalities. Soc Sci Med. 2012;74:236–44. https://doi.org/10.1016/j.socscimed.2011.10.028.

Allport GW. The nature of prejudice. Reading: Addison-Wesley Publishing Company; 1954.

Blum LD. Physicians' goodness and guilt—emotional challenges of practicing medicine. JAMA Intern Med. 2019;179(5):607–8. https://doi.org/10.1001/jamainternmed.2019.0428.

Bourdieu P. The specificity of the scientific field and the social conditions of the progress of reason. Soc Sci Inform. 1975;14(6):19–47. https://doi.org/10.1177/053901847501400602.

Bourdieu P. The forms of capital. In: Richardson J, editor. Handbook of theory and research for the sociology of education. Greenwood: Westport; 1986. p. 241–58.

Bourdieu P. The logic of practice (trans, Nice R). Stanford: Stanford University Press; 1990.

Bourdieu P. Other words (trans, M Adamson). Cambridge: Polity Press; 1994.

Bourdieu P, Wacquant LJD. An invitation to reflexive sociology. Cambridge: Polity Press; 1992.

Buber M. I and thou (trans, R Gregor-Smith). New York: Charles Scribner and Sons; 1937. p. 1958.

Calnan M, Rowe R. Trust relations in a changing health service. J Health Serv Res Policy. 2008;13(3 suppl):97–103. https://doi.org/10.1258/jhsrp.2008.008010.

Charles C, Gafni A, Whelan T. Shared decision-making in the medical encounter: what does it mean (or it takes at least two to tango)? Soc Sci Med. 1997;44(5):681–92. https://doi.org/10.1016/s0277-9536(96)00221-3.

Clark J. Philosophy, understanding and the consultation. Brit J Gen Pract. 2008;58(546):58–60. https://doi.org/10.3399/bjgp08X263929.

Cohen M, Quintner J, Van Rysewyck S. Reconsidering the IASP definition of pain. Pain Rep. 2018;3(2):e634. https://doi.org/10.1097/PR9.0000000000000634.

Cohen ML, Quintner JL, Weisman A. "Nociplastic pain": a challenge to nosology and to nociception. J Pain. 2023;24(12):2131–9. https://doi.org/10.1016/j.pain.2023.07.019.

Cohn S. 'Trust my doctor, trust my pancreas': trust as an emergent quality of social practice. Philos Ethics Humanit Med. 2015;10:1–9. https://doi.org/10.1186/s13010-015-0029-6.

Collyer FM, Willis KF, Franklin M, Harley K, Short SD. Healthcare choice: Bourdieu's capital, habitus and field. Curr Sociol. 2015;63(5):685–99. https://doi.org/10.1177/0011392115590082.

Crisp R. The social brain: how diversity made the modern mind. London: Little, Brown Book Group; 2015. p. 99–112.

Crisp RJ, Turner RN. Imagined intergroup contact. In: Hodson G, Hewstone M, editors. Advances in intergroup contact. Hove: Psychology Press (Taylor and Francis); 2012. p. 135–51.

Duranti A. Husserl, intersubjectivity and anthropology. Anthropol Theory. 2010;10(1):1–20. https://doi.org/10.1177/1463499610370517.

Emmerich N. Medical ethics education: an interdisciplinary and social theoretical perspective. Springer Science and Business Media; 2013. p. 21–39.

Favareau D. Beyond self and other: on the neurosemiotic emergence of intersubjectivity. Sign Syst Stud. 2002;30:57–100. https://doi.org/10.12697/SSS.2002.30.1.05.

Frank AW. "How can they act like that?" clinicians and patients as characters in each other's stories. Hast Cent Rep. 2002;32:14–22.

Frank A. Ethics as process and practice. Int Med J. 2004;34:355–7. https://doi.org/10.1111/j.1445-5994.2004.00622.x.

Glover K. A defense of a monadological analysis in Leibniz's middle years. Aporia. 2008;18(1):13–28.

Gomes AP, Rego S. Pierre Bourdieu and medical education. Rev Bras Educ Med. 2013;37:260–5. https://doi.org/10.1590/S0100-5502201.

Grinnell F. The problem of intersubjectivity: a comparison of Martin Buber and Alfred Schutz. Hum Stud. 1983;6:185–95. https://doi.org/10.1007/BF02127760.

Horton R. Second opinion: doctors, diseases and decisions in modern medicine. London: Granta Books; 2003. p. 1–64.

Husserl E. Cartesian meditations: an introduction to phenomenology. Trans, Dorion Cairns. The Hague: Martinus Nijhoff; 1929. 1960.
Husserl E. In: Kern I, Husserl E, editors. Zur Phänomenologie der Intersubjektivität (on the phenomenology of intersubjectivity). Texts from the *Nachlass*, vol. XV. The Hague: Martinus Nijhoff; 1973. p. 427.
Lyon P, Cohen ML, Quintner JL. An evolutionary stress-response hypothesis for chronic widespread pain (fibromyalgia syndrome). Pain Med. 2011;12:1167–78. https://doi.org/10.1111/j.1526-4637.2011.01168.x.
Matthias MS, Parpart AL, Nyland KA, Huffman MA, Stubbs DL, Sargent C, Blair MJ. The patient-provider relationship in chronic pain: providers' perspective. Pain Med. 2010;11:1688–97. https://doi.org/10.1111/j.1536-4637.2010.00980-x.
Maturana HR, Varela FJ. Autopoiesis and cognition: the realization of the living. Dordecht: Reidel Publishing Co.; 1980.
Maturana HR, Varela FJ. The tree of knowledge. The biological roots of human understanding. Boston: Shambhala; 1987.
Meneses RW, Larkin M. Edith Stein and the contemporary psychological study of empathy. Phenomenol Psychol. 2012;43:151–84. https://doi.org/10.1163/15691624-12341234.
Miles E, Crisp RJ. A meta-analytic test of the imagined contact hypothesis. Group Process Intergroup Relat. 2014;17:3–26. https://doi.org/10.11177/1368430213510573.
Moran D. Edmund Husserl's phenomenon of habituality and habitus. J Br Soc Phenomenol. 2011;42:53–77. https://doi.org/10.1080/00071773.2011.11006731.
Moran D. Edmund Husserl: the crisis of the European sciences and transcendental phenomenology: an introduction. Cambridge: Cambridge University Press; 2012.
Moran D. The phenomenology of the social world: Husserl on *Mitsein* as *Ineinandersein* and *Füreinandersein*. Metodo. 2017;5(1):99–142.
Moran D. From empathy to intersubjectivity: the phenomenological approach. In: Bortolan A, Magrì E, editors. Empathy, intersubjectivity, and the social world: the continued relevance of phenomenology. Essays in Honour of Dermot Moran. Berlin: De Gruyter; 2022. p. 23–44. https://doi.org/10.1515/9783110698787-003.
Navarro Z. In search of a cultural interpretation of power: the contribution of Pierre Bourdieu. IDS Bull. 2006;37(6):11–22.
Nielsen A. Journeys with chronic pain: acquiring stigma along the way. In: McKenzie H, Quintner J, Bendelow G, editors. At the edge of being: the aporia of pain. Oxford: Inter-Disciplinary Press; 2012. p. 83–97.
Overgaard S. What is empathy? In: Kjosavik F, Beyer C, Fricke C, editors. *Husserl's* phenomenology and intersubjectivity: historical interpretations and contemporary applications. New York: Routledge; 2019. p. 178–90.
Owen IR. The significance of Husserl's fifth meditation. Existent Anal. 2000;11(2):11–31.
Praglin L. The nature of the "in-between" in DW Winnicott's concept of the transitional space and in Martin Buber's Zwischenmenschliche. Universitas. 2006;2(2):Article 6.
Pringle R. Sex and medicine: gender, power and Authority in the Medical Profession. Cambridge: Cambridge University Press; 1998. p. 97–127.
Pullman D. Human dignity and the ethics and aesthetics of pain and suffering. Theor Med Bioeth. 2002;23:75–94. https://doi.org/10.1023/a:1019521923979.
Quintner JL, Buchanan D, Cohen ML. Maldynia as a moral judgment. Pain Med. 2011;12:1130. https://doi.org/10.1111/j.1526-4637.2011.01174.x.
Scheler M. The nature of sympathy (transl. Peter heath). London: Routledge and Kegan Paul; 1954.
Stein E. On the problem of empathy. In: Stein W, editor. The collected works of Edith Stein, vol. 3. Washington, DC: ICS Publications; 1917. 1989.
Strasser S. Basic concepts of Edmund Husserl's social ontology. J Philos Res. 1975;29(1):3–33.
Strickland L. The "Monadology". In: Lodge P, Strickland L, editors. Leibniz's key philosophical writings: a guide. Oxford: Oxford University Press; 2020. p. 206–77.

Svenaeus F. The phenomenology of falling ill: an explication, critique and improvement of Sartre's theory of embodiment and alienation. Hum Stud. 2009;32:56–66. https://doi.org/10.1007/s10746-009-9109-1.

Szanto TD. Introduction: empathy and collective intentionality—the social philosophy of Edith Stein. Hum Stud. 2015;38:445–61. https://doi.org/10.1007/s10746-015-9363-3.

Trevarthen C. Pain and mood. In: Wolstenholme G, O'Connor M, editors. Brain and mind, ciba foundation 69. Amsterdam: Excerpta Medica; 1979. p. 23–334.

Varela FJ. In: Di Paolo EA, Thompson E, editors. Principles of biological autonomy. Cambridge, MA: The MIT Press; 2025.

Varela FJ, Thompson E, Rosch E. The embodied mind. Cambridge, MA: The MIT Press; 1991. p. 185–214.

Winnicott DW. Playing and reality. London: Tavistock Publications; 1971.

The Salient Role of Nociception

Abstract Pain in humans—and its analogue in non-verbal animals—is a phenomenon that does not occur without nociception. The function of nociception in signalling to the organism that it has encountered a noxious agent appears to have played a unique role in an evolutionary sense. Although the human "behaviour" of *chronic* pain may appear to be maladaptive, natural selection has favoured mechanisms that respond to tissue damage by increasing the sensitivity of the nociceptive apparatus.

However, the focus of this chapter is not so much on revelations from the biology of nociception but rather on two major epistemological issues. Firstly is the narrowness of the IASP lexicon regarding nociception; secondly, key phenomena have become conflated. Paramount in the latter is the use of "pain descriptors" which are in fact *hypotheses of nociception*. The development of the construct of nociplastic pain has brought this conflation of pain and nociception into focus, exposing the need to reconceptualise both in the interests of maintaining epistemic discipline.

Once the conflations of pain with nociception and of nociplastic pain with central sensitisation of nociception are recognised and resolved, it can be shown that nociception is necessary but not sufficient for pain, which has profound implications for clinical assessment in a biopsychosocial framework and for realigning research activity with clinical aspects, to focus on nociception on the one hand and on distinguishing pain from suffering on the other, with clear therapeutic implications at both individual and public health levels.

A Biological Overview of Nociception

The survival of all animals depends upon their ability to detect harmful ("noxious") stimuli in their environment. By avoiding or minimising bodily harm, they can then prioritise finding sufficient food and reproducing successfully (Burrell 2017).

The detection of noxious stimuli is called *nociception*. In this chapter, it is assigned a *salient* role because it stands out as an attentional event through which organisms learn and survive. It will be argued that nociception is the key to understanding persistent pain. The detection of and response to harmful stimuli involves

M. Cohen, J. Quintner, *A Philosophical Handbook for Pain Medicine Practice*,
https://doi.org/10.1007/978-981-92-1682-6_7

complex physiological processes that appear to have been conserved through evolution (Nesse and Schulkin 2019). The evidence for this can be found at both chemical and behavioural levels in the animal world. Burrell (2017:1461) offers a broad conception: "Nociception represents a critical interaction between an animal and its environment and exhibits considerable evolutionary conservation across species".

Evidence for the Role of Nociception in Natural Selection

Recent insights from the field of evolutionary biology suggest that the pain experience may reflect a "powerful evolutionary adaptation to severe bodily injury" (Walters 2019). Studies in a number of animal groups—fruit flies, molluscs and rodents in particular (Burrell 2017)—indicate that persistent activity of nociceptors has undergone evolutionary selection by being associated with the organism's *survival* long after bodily injury. Survival in this context means more than just continuing to live; it includes avoiding predation and enabling reproduction. It would appear that (persistent) nociceptor activation is a necessary precursor for that survival behaviour in non-human animals which may be analogous to the human pain experience.

Several hypotheses have been proposed to explain why chronic pain in humans is a major clinical problem. One is that the persistent nociceptor hyperactivity that has been demonstrated after bodily injury in a number of different phyla might be an evolutionary adaptive response, in which primitive molecular mechanisms originally related to cellular injury have been repurposed towards facilitating survival (Walters 2019).

We are left with an evolutionary mystery—"why would natural selection shape a regulatory mechanism that expresses pain when it is no longer needed?" (Nesse and Schulkin 2019). A partial explanation is the "fire alarm principle": in signal detection theory, it makes more sense for an alarm to ring loudly when a fire is relatively small than to wait until it has grown large:

> No one would want a smoke detector that almost always detected a fire; we want one that goes off every single time there is a blaze of any kind. To get this reliability, we are willing to accept false alarms. (Nesse 2001:79)

Nociception, as currently understood, performs part of this recognitional function in the face of threats to an organism's structural integrity. Nociception is not the only physiological process that might provide an evolutionary advantage but there is extensive knowledge of its biological basis, including a requirement for a relatively high threshold for activation.

Although the human "behaviour" of *chronic* pain may appear to be maladaptive, natural selection has favoured mechanisms that respond to tissue damage by increasing the sensitivity of the nociceptive apparatus because "the cost of more pain is often vastly less than the cost of too little pain" (Nesse and Schulkin 2019). Pain in humans may therefore be seen as a sensation that would not have emerged without nociception.

Sickness Responses

Nociception can be viewed as protecting an injured organism from expressing behaviours that might interfere with its recovery, thus inducing behaviour appropriate to its survival. Animals in whom nociception is persistent demonstrate sickness responses which appear to be analogous to the human experience of pain after injury (Dantzer et al. 1993; Watkins and Maier 2000). These behaviours include inactivity, aversive responses to non-noxious stimuli, prolonged sleep, depression, as well as disturbances of eating, grooming and social interaction (Dantzer and Kelley 2007). Experimentally induced stress, both in animals and in humans, results in hyperalgesia and allodynia (Crettaz et al. 2013; Jennings et al. 2014). Thus, there appears to be a link between activated stress-response systems, enhanced nociception and sickness behaviour.

On the basis of evidence from diverse disciplines, Lyon et al. (2011) hypothesised that the human experience that is chronic widespread pain (often labelled "fibromyalgia") is one manifestation of persistent activation of an evolutionarily conserved physiological system designed to defend and repair the organism from challenges perceived to threaten its homeostasis.

The Basics of Nociception

Animals possess specialised receptors in body tissues that detect noxious stimuli, coined "nociceptors" by the British neurophysiologist Sir Charles Sherrington (1857–1952) (Sherrington 1906). Nociceptors can be activated by mechanical and chemical stimuli as well as by extremes of environmental temperature. Activation depends upon a variety of ion channels and receptors (Middleton et al. 2021).

Nociceptors have a high threshold for activation, which means they require a relatively large amount of stimulation, in contrast to receptors that register touch, pressure or warm or cool temperature. Nociceptors that respond to combinations of these stimulus types are called "polymodal" (Middleton et al. 2021). Most nociceptive information is carried from nociceptors by specialised nerve fibres (Aδ and C) which synapse onto second-order neurons in the spinal cord. They project upwards to targets in the midbrain, thalamus and cerebrum constituting a very complex system (Coghill 2020). Sherrington coined the term "nociception" for this important process. How these targets process such nociceptive information to result in the pain experience is a "black box" issue that in turn is contingent on consciousness, a topic that is well beyond the scope of this Handbook.

How these basic features may be better conceptualised as a "nociceptive apparatus" will be discussed below.

The Nomenclature of Nociception

Review of Some Pain Terms

In chapter "Clarifying the Definition of Pain", it was argued that the most accurate and parsimonious definition of pain should be "a mutually recognised experience contingent on nociception". It may come as a surprise that, although the term had been in use for a long time, "nociception" was formally defined only in 2008 (Loeser and Treede 2008) and is contained within the current set of definitions adopted by the International Association for the Study of Pain (IASP) (2017). As the potential for confusion is high, commentary on these definitions is offered as footnotes.

The definitions flow as follows:

- noxious stimulus[1]

  1994 version: a noxious stimulus is one that is damaging to normal tissues (Merskey and Bogduk 1994).
  2008 version: a stimulus that is damaging or threatens damage to normal tissues.

- nociceptor

  1994 version: a receptor preferentially sensitive to a noxious stimulus or to a stimulus which would become noxious if prolonged (Merskey and Bogduk 1994).
  2008 version: a high-threshold sensory receptor of the peripheral somatosensory nervous system that is capable of transducing and encoding noxious stimuli.

- nociceptive neuron

  a central or peripheral neuron of the somatosensory nervous system that is capable of encoding noxious stimuli.

  culminating in

[1] It should be noted that "nociceptive stimulus" remains in the taxonomy, defined as "an actually or potentially tissue damaging event transduced and encoded by nociceptors". The first objection is that this hardly differs at all from "a stimulus that is damaging or threatens damage to normal tissues", which is the definition of a noxious stimulus. The second objection is the paradoxical use of the suffix "-ceptive", which is clearly a property of a receptor but here is tied to a stimulus. This leads to the circular argument that a nociceptive stimulus is one that activates nociceptors. But that is what a noxious stimulus does.

- **nociception**[2]

  the neural process of encoding noxious stimuli.

This formulation of nociception focusses solely on the transduction and encoding of a noxious stimulus, that is, on the function of the nociceptor and the (then) newly defined nociceptive neuron. This was a narrowing of previous concepts and attracted critical comment, including the assertion that nociception "should be defined in terms of nervous system responses to noxious stimuli and not in terms of hypothesised responses to a specific afferent type" (Devor 2008). That definitional constraint in turn focussed research on to the structure and function of the nociceptor and nociceptive neuron rather than including any process that might occur after "encoding noxious stimuli".

This would appear to be far too narrow a concept of nociception. In order to develop the argument for a broader reconceptualisation of nociception, it is necessary to revisit so-called "pain descriptors", which in turn will reveal a paradox in terminology that needs to be resolved.

Evolution of "Pain Descriptors"

In chapter "Clarifying the Definition of Pain", it was highlighted that the prime feature in the definition of pain is the linkage with tissue damage, and therefore, by inference, with the signalling of such damage to the organism, namely, "nociception". Most importantly, one of the six Notes that accompany the 2020 definition is "Pain and nociception are different phenomena. Pain cannot be inferred solely from activity in sensory neurons".

However, in contradiction to these statements, the IASP taxonomy contains so-called "pain descriptors", which in fact are *hypotheses of mechanism of nociception.* For some time, two "types" of pain had been informally identified: "nociceptive" and "neuropathic". Surprisingly, a formal definition of "nociceptive pain"—the common-sense or default experience associated with tissue damage—was not the first to be specifically formulated. That distinction fell to "neuropathic pain", defined in 1994 as "pain initiated or caused by a primary lesion or dysfunction in the nervous system" (Merskey and Bogduk 1994). "Dysfunction" of the nervous system was not elaborated upon. Only in 2008 was "nociceptive" pain defined, as that "arising from activation of nociceptors" (Loeser and Treede 2008).

This development established a dichotomy of mechanism: if "activation of nociceptors" by injury or disease could not be established, then "dysfunction" of the nervous system could be presumed. In other words, anything that was not "nociceptive" could be termed "neuropathic".

---

[2] The very term "nociception" implies a process that has been activated. It follows that "activated nociception" is repetitive. By contrast, to talk about "activation of nociceptors", as one mechanism of nociception, is accurate usage.

In 2011, "neuropathic" pain was formally redefined as "Pain caused by a lesion or disease of the somatosensory nervous system" (Jensen et al. 2011). This strict definition not only requires demonstration on clinical or imaging grounds of "a lesion or disease of the somatosensory nervous system"—that is, determination of true neural tissue pathology—but also excludes the concept of "dysfunction".

At that same time,[3] "nociceptive pain" was redefined as "pain that arises from actual or threatened damage to non-neural tissue and is due to activation of nociceptors". This redefinition recapitulated "activation of nociceptors" but limited that to "non-neural" tissue. Furthermore, the Note that accompanies this redefinition states:

> This term is designed to contrast with neuropathic pain. The term is used to describe pain occurring with a normally functioning somatosensory nervous system to contrast with the abnormal function seen in neuropathic pain.

This redefinition perpetuated the "nociceptive–neuropathic" dichotomy as above, but allowed an interpretation that "nociceptive pain" should reflect "a normally functioning somatosensory system", while "neuropathic pain" should reflect "abnormal function" of that system, despite "dysfunction" having been removed from the definition.

It would make biological and linguistic sense to deprecate the use of "pain descriptor" and substitute "mechanism of nociception", so as not to conflate pain and nociception as expressly stated in the Note to the 2020 definition of pain. Because of established usage, that is unlikely to happen. However, "nociceptive pain" could be redefined simply as "pain caused by activation of nociceptors".[4] This common-sense biological position presumes that the tissue was "normal" before encountering the noxious stimulus and that the somatosensory apparatus is also "normal". The definition of "neuropathic pain" would remain robust, as "pain caused by a lesion or disease of the somatosensory nervous system".

In this context, it is worth pointing out that the Note that accompanies the definition of "neuropathic pain" states "Neuropathic pain is a clinical description (and not a diagnosis)". The same admonition applies to "nociceptive pain" and, as will be shown, to "nociplastic pain".

The Need for a Third "Descriptor"

Although the 2011 redefinition of neuropathic pain made biological and etymological sense, it left out a large group of patients whose pain could not then attract either "nociceptive" or "neuropathic" as a "pain descriptor". Many of these patients had

---

[3] It should be mentioned that 2011 remains the most recent iteration of the nociceptive and neuropathic "descriptors". The third "descriptor"—nociplastic—was not added until 2017.

[4] Strictly speaking, that should be "pain caused by nociceptive nociception", which sounds strange and would be confusing. Similarly, "neuropathic pain" should be "pain caused by neuropathic nociception".

conditions such as those currently labelled as fibromyalgia, complex regional pain syndrome, "non-specific" chronic low back pain, irritable bowel syndrome and other "functional" visceral pain disorders. Prior to the redefinition, these conditions would have been attributed to "dysfunction" of the nervous system and therefore would have fallen under the "neuropathic" rubric. In these conditions, there is neither obvious activation of nociceptors nor evidence of neuropathy (as defined by the IASP). Yet patients with these conditions present with clinical features which suggest that nociception has occurred, as typically they are characterised by (a) pain in a regional or more widespread distribution and (b) clinical and elicitable hypersensitivity, including allodynia, in apparently normal tissues. The phenomena in (b) lead to an inescapable inference that a change from normal nociceptive function has occurred.

These considerations demanded that a third descriptor be developed, to cater for these cases that now fell into a state of uncertainty in terms of mechanism of nociception. In November 2017, the IASP adopted "nociplastic pain", formally defined as,

> Pain that arises from altered nociception despite no clear evidence of actual or threatened tissue damage causing the activation of peripheral nociceptors or evidence for disease or lesion of the somatosensory system causing the pain. (Kosek et al. 2016)

More simply, "nociplastic" pain is attributed to "altered nociception" but is neither "nociceptive" nor "neuropathic". The original publication referred to the key concept of evidence of *altered nociception*—essentially allodynia to certain stimuli—related to ostensibly normal tissue in a region of pain (Kosek et al. 2016). In retrospect, it is not so much that nociception is altered, rather that it has been engaged by one or more processes that are neither "nociceptive" nor "neuropathic" (Cohen et al. 2023).

The intention here was threefold: to confer validity on the pain experience in those patient groups and thus avoid potentially stigmatising labels such as "pathological", "dysfunctional", "idiopathic" and "unexplained"; to facilitate communication between patients, clinicians and other stakeholder groups; and to stimulate clinical and basic discussion and research into the phenomena of altered nociceptive function, with the ultimate goal of developing new treatment strategies.

Reactions to the Construct of "Nociplastic" Pain

The construct of "nociplastic pain" continues to be met with divergent receptions. On the one hand, it has been enthusiastically embraced, to the extent of conflation with "primary" pain (ICD-11; see chapter "The Non-Convergent Language Used in Clinical and Taxonomic Settings") and with central sensitisation of nociception as well as the promulgation of "nociplastic pain syndromes", which will be discussed in detail below.

For the moment, the focus will be on the rejection of the construct by those whose scepticism derives from the absence, according to the definition above, of underlying activation of nociceptors (Loeser 2022). In contrast to Sherrington's integrative view of nociception, as described above, the current definition focussed research on identifying the structure and function of the "nociceptor" and the (newly defined) "nociceptive neuron". The only IASP definition that refers to any process that might occur after "the neural process of encoding noxious stimuli" is that of "central sensitisation of nociception".[5]

The question then arises, in view of the phenomena that nociplastic pain seeks to address, is such a narrow conception still tenable?

"Nociplastic Pain" Exposes the Inadequacy of Nociception as Currently Defined

The twin IASP definitions of nociception as "the neural process of encoding noxious stimuli" and of a noxious stimulus as one that is "damaging or threatens damage to normal tissues" can be amalgamated to denote "nociception-as-currently-defined (NACD)". NACD then posits that nociception relates *only* to the recognition of a noxious stimulus via nociceptors, defined in the singular as "a high-threshold sensory receptor of the peripheral somatosensory nervous system that is capable of transducing and encoding noxious stimuli".

Viewed through this lens, the construct of "nociplastic" pain does indeed describe an experience that occurs in the absence of NACD. However, it nonetheless accords with the definition of pain to the extent that it resembles an experience that is associated with NACD. That resemblance is phenotypically indistinguishable from the situation when NACD has been "activated". It seems, therefore, reasonable to postulate that a process which may be associated with pain has been activated other than via nociceptors: hence the inferred "altered nociception" or "altered nociceptive function"[6] (Cohen et al. 2023).

This also highlights a paradox in the definition of pain that was discussed in chapter "Clarifying the Definition of Pain": that nociplastic pain denotes an experience that occurs in the absence of NACD, which contradicts the definition of pain, while simultaneously nociplastic pain is consistent with the definition of pain to the extent that it resembles an experience that is associated with NACD.

This paradox can be resolved in one of three ways: by redefining pain, by redefining nociception or by redefining both these terms.

In chapter "Clarifying the Definition of Pain", it was proposed that pain be redefined as "an unpleasant sensory and emotional experience contingent on

[5] This is defined as "increased responsiveness of nociceptive neurons in the central nervous system to their normal or subthreshold afferent input" and will be discussed below.

[6] It could be argued that this "altered nociception" is, in fact, "nociceptive dysfunction".

nociception"—or, preferably, "a mutually recognised experience contingent on nociception"—with the caveat that NACD be reconceptualised (Cohen et al. 2026). This discussion now turns to the proposal that nociception be redefined as activation of a nociceptive apparatus.

Nociceptive System or Apparatus

Description

Sherrington's ground-breaking work culminated in the concept of a nociceptive system (Sherrington 1920:345), which has been revisited in recent years as a "distributed nociceptive system" (Coghill 2020) and a "nociceptive apparatus" (Cohen et al. 2023).

Invertebrates and vertebrates possess segregated sensory pathways within the nervous system dedicated to the transmission of nociceptive information. They are widely distributed, allowing different elements to perform the same function (Coghill 2020). This ensures the adaptability of nociception and its ability to maintain functionality even when some of its components are disrupted. These properties explain the failure of many attempts to relieve pain by cutting relevant nerves and their pathways within the body (Willis and Westlund 1997) (Fig. 1).

This figure illustrates the structural and functional organisation of the nociceptive apparatus at peripheral, spinal and supraspinal levels.

Peripheral Components

The peripheral aspect of the apparatus has two distinct branches of nociceptive neurons, both containing Aδ and C fibre populations (Picture 1). The red dots indicate chemical mediators/cytokines that initiate nociception, directly in a region of tissue damage (left) or released from immune system cells (right). The superficial branch of the nociceptive neuron innervates cutaneous nociceptors that can be activated by local noxious thermal, mechanical and chemical stimuli (Picture 2). The deep branch innervates nociceptors in muscles and joints that can be activated by noxious mechanical stimuli, and in viscera that can be activated by noxious distension (Picture 3). The cell bodies of both branches of these nociceptive neurons reside in the dorsal root ganglion. Their central projections enter the posterior horn of the spinal cord, where they synapse with second-order nociceptive neurons.

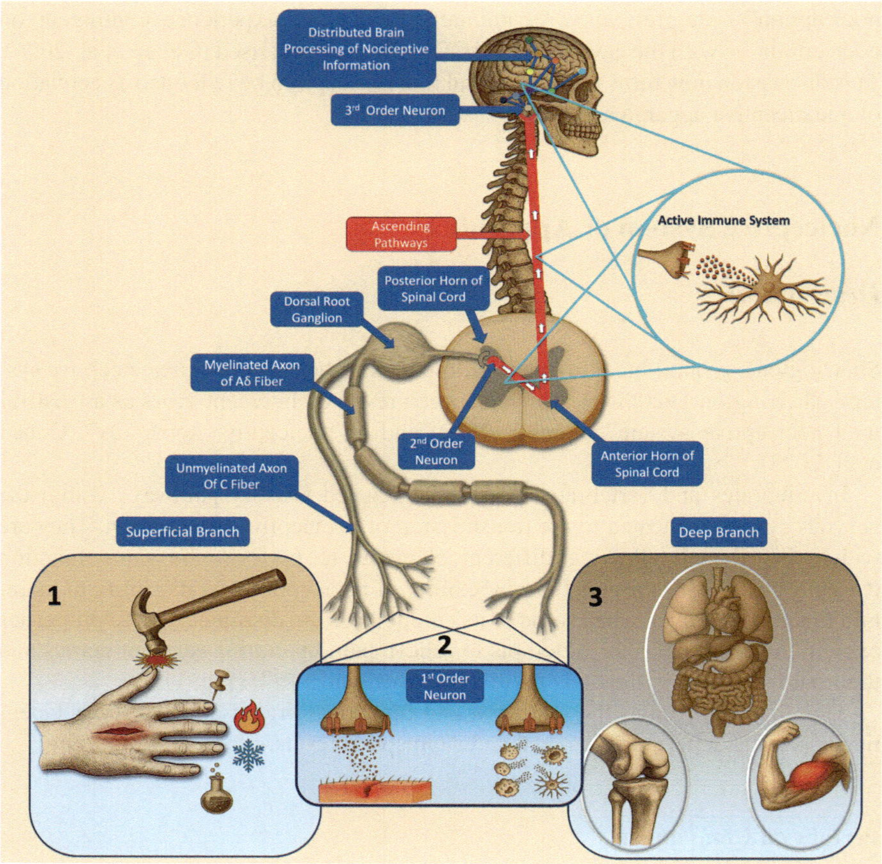

Fig. 1 The nociceptive apparatus: peripheral, central and immune components. (Courtesy of Dr. Asaf Weisman, with permission)

Central Components

After synapsing in the posterior horn, second-order neurons cross to the contralateral side of the spinal cord and ascend primarily through the anterior and lateral spinothalamic pathways. These tracts convey nociceptive information that is integrated in distributed brain regions responsible for sensory discrimination, affective responses and cognitive evaluation. Third-order neurons in supraspinal structures complete the sequence from peripheral detection to central representation, integrating neural and immune-derived signals.

Chemical Basis

In the spinal cord and the brain, the immune system influences the processes of nociception. Glial cells, peripherally and residing in the central nervous system itself, including macrophages, microglia, astrocytes and infiltrating leucocytes, generate signalling molecules that modulate synaptic transmission of nociceptive input.

Modulation of Nociceptive Function

"Switch-Off": Inhibition of Nociception

The function of the ascending pathways that carry nociceptive information to the brain can be inhibited by substances originating elsewhere in the body, especially from the immune system. This arrangement allows for the necessary dynamic changes in threshold for nociception in accordance with the organism's priorities at the time (Heinricher et al. 2008).

"Switch-On": Sensitisation of Nociception

In biology, "sensitisation" refers to a state of increased responsiveness to a stimulus. In neurophysiology, sensitisation is characterised by a decreased threshold for discharge and/or increased amplitude of activity of nerves, in this case nociceptive pathways (Sandkühler 2009). In simple terms, peripheral and central sensitisation of nociception can be thought of as physiological increase in function of the nociceptive apparatus.

(a) *Peripheral Sensitisation of Nociception*

Activation of nociceptors in response to a noxious stimulus is usually but not always associated with a pain experience. Activated nociceptors may become sensitised such that they discharge in response to non-noxious stimulation (Sandkühler 2009).

This is the common experience of "tenderness": the part hurts—it is "painful"—when it is touched or moved gently—that is, subjected to a non-noxious stimulus. Technically, this phenomenon is called *allodynia* (literally, "other pain") (IASP 1994). Other examples of allodynia include pain from clothing brushing against the skin or from a cold breeze blowing onto skin. Clearly, these stimuli are not noxious, so something has happened to the nociceptors such that they discharge and may lead to a pain experience: they have become sensitised.

(b) *Central Sensitisation of Nociception*

This neurophysiological process of sensitisation can also involve nociceptive pathways within the central nervous system. The phenomenon has been demonstrated in many different species but can only be inferred from clinical signs in humans. Central sensitisation of nociception occurs when spinal cord nociceptive neurons have been subjected to repeated episodes of noxious input from the relevant peripheral nerves (Sandkühler 2009; Woolf 1983). These neurons also become sensitised when exposed to various products released by nearby activated glial cells, which are now known to be part of the immune system (Ren and Dubner 2008).

The spinal cord dorsal horn is a major site for experiments that may induce and maintain pain behaviour in animals in response to non-noxious mechanical stimuli (mechanical allodynia). Local circuits within the network allow low-threshold mechanosensory fibres to access nociceptive neurons (Peirs et al. 2021). Additionally, in this model, direct cortical modulation of normal and pathological tactile sensory processing in the spinal cord via descending supraspinal neurons projecting to the deep dorsal horn has been shown (Liu et al. 2018).

Underpinning this role of spinal dorsal horn neurons as a major relay for nociceptive information are substance P (SP) and related tachykinins that are also involved in very many other neuronal signalling pathways, including sensations and emotional responses (Zeiglgänsberger 2019). SP is released from primary afferent fibres following noxious input and excites nociceptive neurons in the dorsal horn of the spinal cord. It is also expressed by a variety of non-neuronal cell types such as microglia, as well as immune cells, such as T cells, tissue-resident macrophages, dendritic cells and eosinophils. In rodent experiments, spinal neurons expressing the substance-P-receptor are required for the development and maintenance of central sensitisation of nociception and hyperalgesia (Khasabov et al. 2002).

Avoiding Conflation of Concepts

Conflation of Pain and Nociception

Conflation, a major theme in this Handbook, is a fallacy that occurs when distinct things are treated as if they were the same. In the literature, pain and nociception are all too frequently conflated (see also chapters "Trying to Gain Traction on a Slippery Subject", "Errors in Language and Logic Call for Epistemic Discipline" and "Case Studies in Tautology, Circular Reasoning and Conflation: Fibromyalgia and Myofascial Pain "Syndromes""), despite the Note to the 2020 iteration of the IASP definition of pain that states, "Pain and nociception are different phenomena. Pain cannot be inferred solely from activity in sensory neurons" (see chapter "Clarifying the Definition of Pain").

Nociception is the signalling to the organism that bodily damage has occurred. However, nociception is not always associated with a pain experience. For example, a soldier injured in the heat of battle may not have a pain experience until much later (Beecher 1956). In causal language, this means that nociception is not sufficient for pain.

Pain, certainly in humans, is a complex response that is driven by nociception in the first instance but may be modified by many other factors. This has generated *biopsychosocial conceptual frameworks* in which nociception is the dimension of what is happening to the body. In addition to this, there is also what is happening to the person, labelled the "psychological" dimension and what is happening in the persons' world, labelled the "social" dimension (see chapter "Conceptual Frameworks"). It is also why the correct terminology is "nociceptive" nerves and pathways, not "pain" nerves and pathways (see chapter "Errors in Language and Logic Call for Epistemic Discipline").

Conflation of Nociplastic Pain and Central Sensitisation of Nociception

Following the promulgation of "nociplastic" pain, many who had championed the concept of "centralized" pain adopted it in name but used it as a synonym for "central sensitization". A typical, clear example of such conflation is demonstrated in this statement:

> CS [central sensitization] is not part of the definition of nociplastic pain; however, signs of sensitization are generally present in nociplastic pain conditions. Moreover, sensitization is the major underlying mechanism of nociplastic pain. Hence, patients whose clinical picture is dominated by CS are labelled as having nociplastic pain. (Nijs et al. 2021a)

It seems important, therefore, to distinguish "central sensitisation", which is a neurophysiological phenomenon, from "nociplastic pain" which is used as a "clinical descriptor" although technically that is a misnomer[7] (Cohen et al. 2023). Firstly, it is necessary to consider again the IASP definition of "central sensitisation (of nociception)", namely, "increased responsiveness of nociceptive neurons in the central nervous system to their normal or subthreshold afferent input" (IASP 2017). This is a phenomenon that cannot be demonstrated *in vivo* in humans. This caveat leads to consideration of two contemporary conceptualisations of "central sensitisation":

- … we define central sensitisation as an amplification of neural signalling within the CNS that elicits pain hypersensitivity (Nijs et al. 2021b); and
- Central sensitization is a physiological concept that has been recognized as a generator of pain hypersensitivity by central neural plasticity. (Treede et al. 2019).

Both these statements feature circular argument, summarised as "central sensitisation" is a "central" neural process of "amplification" or "plasticity". More importantly, what precisely is meant by "pain hypersensitivity?"[8] As has been argued in chapter "Clarifying the Definition of Pain", pain is not a "thing" to which an organism can be sensitive, insensitive or hypersensitive (Cohen et al. 2023). In the litera-

---

[7] See discussion in chapter "Errors in Language and Logic Call for Epistemic Discipline".

[8] Ibid.

ture, "pain sensitivity" is shorthand for "sensitivity to pain", implying that pain is a stimulus. But pain is, by definition, an experience, that is, a response; being "sensitive" is also a response. An organism cannot be "sensitive" to its own response. If, as it seems, by "pain hypersensitivity" these authors (and others) wish to denote an increased pain experience in response to a defined stimulus, then it is *engaged nociception* to which they are referring, as a possible result of "amplification" or "plasticity". In other words, the phenomenon under consideration is central sensitisation *of nociception*, not "pain hypersensitivity".

This emphasis on central sensitisation *of nociception* above is important, as some authors have taken the conflation further, for example:

> Central sensitisation goes beyond the nociceptive system and pain experience. It is key for clinicians to understand *that non-pain symptoms can result from the same underlying mechanism* (i.e., central sensitisation). (Nijs et al. 2021a) (Emphasis added here.)

The assertion in italics is conjecture: given the definitional association of pain with tissue damage/nociception (chapter "Clarifying the Definition of Pain"), there is no *a priori* reason for any "non-pain" symptoms to be associated with nociception, quite apart from there being no mechanistic evidence for such a claimed association.

Nothing in this discussion denies the possibility that central sensitisation of nociception may well be an important mechanism that underlies clinically determined "nociplastic pain", once criteria have been sufficiently validated, given that only indirect inference is possible in humans. It is a working hypothesis that needs to be considered alongside others such as somatic hypervigilance.

Conflation of "Nociplastic" Pain and "Primary" Pain

Others authors (Fitzcharles et al. 2021) have taken conflation further, by inviting the reader down a path where "chronic primary pain"[9] implies "nociplastic pain" which in turn implies "central sensitisation of nociception", despite the differences identified above between a taxonomic entity, a descriptor of pain (hypothesis of nociception) and an underlying neurophysiological mechanism.

These same authors assert not only that "nociplastic pain" is a diagnosis-in-its-own-right but also that it can account for all conditions "that cannot be better accounted for by another chronic pain condition", which happens to be the main criterion for "chronic primary pain". In the absence of validated clinical criteria and clinicopathological correlations for identifying nociplastic pain (Kosek et al. 2021; Cohen 2022a, b), such a claim is premature. However, Fitzcharles et al. (2021) assert further that nociplastic pain "encompasses symptoms beyond pain", which leads them to describe "categories" of "nociplastic pain syndromes", an extrapolation that verges on the tautological as they are said to account for

[9] See chapter "The Non-Convergent Language Used in Clinical and Taxonomic Settings".

> … pain conditions that are neither neuropathic nor nociceptive, are real but difficult to diagnose, and commonly experienced by persons worldwide.

But how can a descriptor for a mechanism of nociception encompass "symptoms beyond pain"?

A recently published field study has illustrated the pitfalls of this conflation (Schmidt et al. 2025). Suggested criteria for nociplastic pain (Kosek et al. 2021) were applied to 52 patients with "chronic primary pain": 40% (95%CI 27–53%) failed to meet those criteria. This is not unexpected, given that taxonomic and physiological criteria were being compared. However, the issue was found to turn on the "hypersensitivity" phenomena—that is, allodynia[10] (Cohen 2022a, b; Cohen et al. 2025) (Table 1).

Table 1 Distinguishing between central sensitisation of nociception, nociplastic pain and primary pain

	Central sensitisation of nociception	Nociplastic pain	Primary pain
Field	Neurophysiology	Clinical medicine	Taxonomy
Focus	Neuronal function	Clinical description	Coding
Tool(s)	(a) Direct neural interrogation (b) Psychophysical inference	Clinical inference (elicitation of hyperaesthetic phenomena)	Definition
Amenable to experimental demonstration	Yes	No	N/A
Concept	(a) Use-dependent synaptic plasticity in spinal cord (b) Others	"Clinical descriptor"[a] for pain that is: (i) not nociceptive or neuropathic; and (ii) associated with allodynia elicited in region of pain	Pain as a condition in its own right
Mechanism—*demonstrated*	Long-term potentiation[b]	Not yet established	Agnostic
Mechanism—*hypothesised*: (a) Conceptual or system level	Deficient endogenous pain modulation[c]	Altered central nociceptive function; increased activity of central nociceptive apparatus	Agnostic
Mechanism—*hypothesised*: (b) Granular or tissue level	Neuroinflammatory processes (glial/neuronal interaction)	Agnostic	Agnostic
Diagnostic entity	No	No	Equivocal[d]

(continued)

[10] As discussed in chapter "Translation into the Clinic".

Table 1 (continued)

	Central sensitisation of nociception	Nociplastic pain	Primary pain
Clinical recognition	Inference only[e]	Yes (although definitive criteria yet to be determined[e,f])	Yes ("... cannot be better accounted for by another chronic pain condition"[f,g]).

Modified from Cohen et al. (2023)
Notes:
[a]As argued in this handbook, the term "pain descriptor" is strictly a misnomer, as the adjectives used—nociceptive, neuropathic and nociplastic—denote hypotheses of nociception, not pain experiences
[b]Klein et al. (2008)
[c]See chapter "Errors in Language and Logic Call for Epistemic Discipline" for discussion of "pain modulation"
[d]See chapter "The Non-Convergent Language Used in Clinical and Taxonomic Settings"
[e]Central sensitisation in humans cannot be determined, according to the IASP definition, as input is not possible.
[f]See chapter "Translation into the Clinic"
[g]Nicholas et al. (2019)

Nociception as Necessary but Not Sufficient for Pain

In chapter "Clarifying the Definition of Pain", it was shown that the current definition of pain can be reformulated, without any compromise of its intent, as "Pain is an unpleasant sensory and emotional experience associated with nociception", or preferably revised to "an unpleasant sensory and emotional experience contingent on nociception", or even further to "a mutually recognised experience contingent on nociception", with the vital caveat that nociception itself needs to be redefined (Cohen et al. 2026).

Given that pain and nociception are different phenomena, what is the connection between them? There are abundant examples of individuals sustaining tissue damage (and therefore probably incurring nociception) without reporting pain (Del Rosso et al. 2006; Volmer-Thole and Lobman 2016). This uncontroversial phenomenon is captured by the assertion that "nociception can occur without pain", which can be rephrased as "nociception is not sufficient for pain". However, it is commonly coupled with another assertion, that "pain can occur without nociception", which can be rephrased as "nociception is not necessary for pain". These two assertions have been incorporated into a popular aphorism,[11] "nociception is neither necessary nor sufficient for pain" (Tracey 2005; Moseley and Vlaeyen 2015), which is pervasive in the literature and seemingly accepted as established knowledge (Weisman et al. 2026).

[11]An aphorism is a short saying that is intended to express a general truth.

However, there is a logical contradiction between the first assertion in this aphorism—nociception is not necessary for pain—and the connection between pain and nociception implied by the IASP definition as it stands and in its evolved forms. In other words, the definition in essence requires that if pain is present then nociception has occurred.

It has recently been shown that there is no empirical clinical or experimental evidence that confidently supports the proposition that pain can arise without actual activation of peripheral or central spinal cord neurons responsible for nociception (Weisman et al. 2026).

What follows logically from *operationally* reframing the definition as "an unpleasant sensory and emotional experience contingent on nociception" is that the presence of pain implies that nociception-in-some-form has been engaged. This means that any assertion that pain can arise spontaneously is incompatible with that definition.

The biological argument has two aspects. The first is the evolutionary advantage conferred on organisms that have a mechanism for recognising if not also responding to allostatic load, as discussed earlier in this Chapter. The second aspect is the absence of plausible empirical evidence that the pain experience, as defined and mutually understood, does occur without nociception-in-some-form or, to put that another way, the lack of evidence that pain can arise spontaneously.

Thus, from both logical and biological points of view, the assertion that nociception is not necessary for pain is unsustainable. As such, the aphorism should be revised to "nociception is necessary but not sufficient for pain" (Weisman et al. 2026).

Implications of Reconceptualising Nociception

The implications of reconceptualising nociception are profound. Acceptance of the necessity of nociception for pain, in a new paradigm of activation of a nociceptive apparatus, has two major sets of sequelae. The first is that all pain, especially chronic pain, is potentially explainable at a biological (somatic) level. This makes untenable the view that non-somatic factors—psychological or social—cause pain, because they do not involve nociception**.** In other words, psychological and/or social factors are neither necessary nor sufficient for a pain experience. This does not deny the influence of such factors on modifying that pain experience or the importance of considering these dimensions on a par with the "biological" or somatic dimension in a clinical biopsychosocial conceptual framework.[12]

The second implication is that the metaphorical use of "pain" to denote suffering can be parsed according to whether or not that complaint is attributable to nociception. This distinction has only recently come under closer scrutiny, as discussed in chapter "Trying to Gain Traction on a Slippery Subject". Not all pain experiences

[12] See also chapter "Conceptual Frameworks".

are necessarily associated with suffering and not all suffering in a person experiencing pain may be due to nociception. This also has major clinical implications, as it is incumbent upon the health professional not only to recognise suffering but also to determine to what that might be attributable. Not all complaints of "pain" may have a somatic origin but an expanded concept of nociception would confer validation for many of those people whose pain is often labelled as "medically unexplained". This is in fact embraced in the recent construct of "nociplastic" pain, which is not a label of exclusion but requires clinical evidence that suggests that nociception has been engaged in the absence of "nociceptive" or "neuropathic" processes.

Thus, the principle captured by the revised aphorism, "nociception is necessary but not sufficient for pain", can be seen to fundamentally reset clinical assessment of the somatic (or "biological") dimension of the biopsychosocial framework and the therapeutic approaches to that, without detracting at all from the importance of the psychological and social dimensions. This would also serve to realign research activity with clinical aspects, to focus on nociception on the one hand and on distinguishing pain from suffering on the other, with clear therapeutic implications at both individual and public health levels (Weisman et al. 2026).

References

Beecher HK. Relationship of significance of wound to pain experienced. JAMA. 1956;161(17):1609–13. https://doi.org/10.1001/jama.1956.02970170005002.

Burrell BD. Comparative biology of pain: what invertebrates can tell us about how nociception works. J Neurophysiol. 2017;117(4):1461–73. https://doi.org/10.1152/jn.00600.2016.

Coghill RC. The distributed nociceptive system—a framework for understanding pain. Trends Neurosci. 2020;43(10):780–94. https://doi.org/10.1016/j.tins.2020.07.004.

Cohen ML. Proposed clinical criteria for nociplastic pain in the musculoskeletal system are flawed. Pain. 2022a;163:e606–7. https://doi.org/10.1097/j.pain.0000000000002505.

Cohen ML. Clarifying "chronic primary musculoskeletal pain"? The waters remain murky. Invited Comment Pain Rep. 2022b;7:e1021. https://doi.org/10.1097/PR9.0000000000001021.

Cohen M, Quintner J, Weisman A. "Nociplastic pain": a challenge to nosology and nociception. J Pain. 2023;24(12):2131–9. https://doi.org/10.1016/j.jpain.2023.07.019.

Cohen M, Quintner J, Weisman A. "Primary" and "nociplastic" pain must not be conflated. Pain. 2025;156:1949–50. https://doi.org/10.1097/j.pain.0000000000003659.

Cohen ML, Weisman A, Quintner JL. Paradoxes weaken the IASP definition of pain. Korean J Pain. 2026;39(1):1–8. https://doi.org/10.3344/kjp.25268.

Crettaz B, Marziniak M, Willeke P, Young P, Hellhammer D, Stumpf A, Burgmer M. Stress-induced allodynia—evidence of increased pain sensitivity in healthy humans and patients with chronic pain after experimentally induced psychosocial stress. PLoS One. 2013;8:e69460. https://doi.org/10.1371/journal.pone.0069460.

Dantzer R, Kelley KW. Twenty years of research into cytokine-induced sickness behavior. Brain Behav Immun. 2007;21(2):153–60. https://doi.org/10.1016/j.bbi.09.006.

Dantzer R, Bluthe R, Kent S, Goodall G. Behavioral effects of cytokines: an insight into mechanisms of sickness behavior. In: De Souza EB, editor. Neurobiology of cytokines, Volume 17, Part B. La Jolla: Neurocrine Biosciences, Inc; 1993. p. 130–50. https://doi.org/10.1016/S1043-9471(13)70013-2.

Del Rosso A, Matucci Cerinic M, De Giorgio F, Minari C, Maria Rotella C, Seghieri G. Rheumatological manifestations in diabetes mellitus. Curr Diabetes Res. 2006;2(4):455–66. https://doi.org/10.2174/157339981060204045 5.

Devor M. Nociception in Kyoto. Pain. 2008;140:519–20. https://doi.org/10.1016/j.pain.2008.09.012.

Fitzcharles MS, Cohen SP, Clauw DJ, Littlejohn G, Usui C, Haüser W. Nociplastic pain: towards an understanding of prevalent pain conditions. Lancet. 2021;397(10289):2098–110. https://doi.org/10.1016/S0140-6736(21)00392-5.

Heinricher MM, Ingram SL. The brainstem and nociceptive modulation. Pain 2008;5:593–626. https://doi.org/10.1016/B978-012370880-9.00183-5.

IASP. Pain terms, a current list with definitions and notes on usage. In: Merskey H, Bogduk N, editors. IASP task force on taxonomy. Classification of pain, 2nd ed. Seattle: IASP Press, 1994: 209–214.

International Association for the Study of Pain (IASP). IASP Terminology 2017. Available from: https://www.iasp-pain.org/terminology?navItemNumber=576

Jennings EM, Okine BN, Roche M, Finn DP. Stress-induced hyperalgesia. Prog Neurobiol. 2014;121:1–18. https://doi.org/10.1016/j.pneurobio.2014.06.03.

Jensen TS, Baron R, Haanpaa M, et al. A new definition of neuropathic pain. Pain. 2011;152:2204–5. https://doi.org/10.1016/j.pain.2011.06.017.

Khasabov SG, Rogers SD, Ghilardi JR, Peters CM, Mantyh PW, Simone DA. Spinl neurons that possess the substance P receptor are required for the development of central sensitization. J Neurosci. 2002;22(20):9086–98. https://doi.org/10.1523/JNEUROSCI.22-20-09086.2002.

Klein T, Stahn S, Magerl W, Treede R-D. The role of heterosynaptic facilitation in Long-term potentiation (LTP) of human pain sensation. Pain. 2008;139:507–19.

Kosek E, Cohen M, Baron R, Gebhart GF, Mico J-A, Rice ASC, et al. Do we need a third mechanistic descriptor for chronic pain states? Pain. 2016;157(7):1382–6. j.pain.0000000000000507

Kosek E, Clauw D, Nijs J, et al. Chronic nociplastic pain affecting the musculoskeletal system: clinical criteria and grading system. Pain. 2021;162:2629–34. https://doi.org/10.1097/j.pain.00000000000023242639-2634.

Liu Y, Latremoliere A, Li X, Zhang Z, Chen M, Wang X, Fang C, Alexander C, Gao Z, Chew B, Ding X, Zhou J-Y, Zhang Y, Chen C, Wank KH, Woolf CJ, He Z. Touch and tactile neuropathic pain sensitivity are set by corticospinal projections. Nature. 2018;561(7724):547–50. https://doi.org/10.1038/s41586-018-0515-2.

Loeser JD. A new way of thinking about pain. Pain. 2022;163(9):1670–4. https://doi.org/10.1097/j.pain.0000000000002583.

Loeser JD, Treede R-D. The Kyoto protocol of IASP basic pain terminology. Pain. 2008;137(3):473–7. https://doi.org/10.1016/j.pain.2008.04.025.

Lyon P, Cohen ML, Quintner JL. An evolutionary stress-response hypothesis for chronic widespread pain (fibromyalgia syndrome). Pain Med. 2011;12:1167–78. https://doi.org/10.1111/j.1526-4637.2011.01168.x.

Merskey H, Bogduk N, editors. Classification of chronic pain. 2nd ed. Seattle: IASP Press; 1994.

Middleton SJ, Barry AM, Comini M, Li Y, Ray PR, Shiers S, et al. Studying human nociceptors: from fundamentals to clinic. Brain. 2021;144:1312–35. https://doi.org/10.1093/brain/awab048.

Moseley GL, Vlaeyen JWS. Beyond nociception: the imprecision hypothesis of pain. Pain. 2015;156(1):35–8. https://doi.org/10.1016/j.pain.0000000000000014.

Nesse RM. The smoke detector principle: natural selection and the regualtion of defense responses. Ann N Y Acad Sci. 2001;935(1):75–85. https://doi.org/10.1111/j.1749-6632.2001.tb03472.x.

Nesse RM, Schulkin J. An evolutionary medicine perspective on pain and its disorders. Philos Trans R Soc B. 2019;374(1785):20190288. https://doi.org/10.1098/rstb.2019.0288.

Nicholas M, Vlaeyen JWS, Rief W, Barke A, Aziz Q, Benoliel R, Cohen M, Evers S, Giamberardino MA, Goebel A, Korwisi B, Perrot S, Svensson P, Wang S-J, Treede R-D. The IASP classification of chronic pain for ICD-11: chronic primary pain. Pain. 2019;160:28–37. https://doi.org/10.1097/j.pain.0000000000001390.

Nijs J, Lahousse A, Kapreli E, Bilika P, Saraçoğlu İ, Malfliet A, Coppieters I, De Baets L, Leysen L, Roose E, Clark J, Voogt L, Huysmans E. Nociplastic pain criteria or recognition of central sensitization? Pain phenotyping in the past, present and future. J Clin Med. 2021a;10(15):3203. https://doi.org/10.3390/jcm10153203.

Nijs J, George SZ, Clauw DJ, Fernaández-de-Las-Peñas C, Kosek E, et al. Central sensitisation in chronic pain conditions: latest discoveries and their potential for precision medicine. Lancet Rheumatol. 2021b;3(5):e392. https://doi.org/10.1016/S2665-9913(21)00032-1.

Peirs C, Williams S-PG, Zhao X, Arokiaraj CM, Ferreira DW, Noh M-c, Smith KM, Halder P, Corrigan KA, et al. Mechanical allodynia circuitry in the dorsal horn is defined by the nature of the injury. Neuron. 2021;109:73–90. https://doi.org/10.1016/j.neuron.2020.10.027.

Ren K, Dubner R. Neuron–glia crosstalk gets serious: role in pain hypersensitivity. Curr Opin Anesthesiol. 2008;21(5):570–9. https://doi.org/10.1097/ACO.0b013e32830edbdf.

Sandkühler J. Models and mechanisms of hyperalgesia and allodynia. Physiol Rev. 2009;89:707–58. https://doi.org/10.1152/physrev.00025.2008.

Schmidt H, Drusko A, Renz MP, Schlömp L, Tost H, Schuh-Hofer S, et al. Application of the grading system for "nociplastic pain" in chronic primary and chronic secondary pain conditions: a field study. Pain. 2025;166(1):196–211. https://doi.org/10.1097/j.pain.0000000000003355.

Sherrington CS. The integrative action of the nervous system. London: Archibald Constable and Co.; 1906.

Sherrington CS. The integrative action of the nervous system. New Haven: Yale University Press; 1920.

Tracey I. Nociceptive processing in the human brain. Curr Opin Neurobiol. 2005;15(4):478–87. https://doi.org/10.1016/j.conb.2005.06.010.

Treede R-D, Rief W, Barke A, Aziz Q, Bennett MI, Benoliel R, et al. Chronic pain as a symptom or a disease: the IASP classification of chronic pain for the International Classification of Diseases (ICD-11). Pain. 2019;160(1):19–27. https://doi.org/10.1097/j.pain.0000000000001384.

Volmer-Thole M, Lobman R. Neuropathy and diabetic foot syndrome. Int J Mol Sci. 2016;17(6):917. https://doi.org/10.3390/ijms17060917.

Walters ET. Adaptive mechanisms driving maladaptive pain: how chronic ongoing activity in primary nociceptors can enhance evolutionary fitness after severe injury. Philos Trans R Soc B. 2019;347:20190277. https://doi.org/10.1098/rstb.2019.0277.

Watkins LR, Maier SF. The pain of being sick: implications of immune-to-brain communiction for understanding pain. Annu Rev Psychol. 2000;51:29–57. https://doi.org/10.1146/annurev.psych.51.29.

Weisman AK, Quintner JL, Cohen ML. Adieu to an aphorism: nociception is necessary for pain. Brain. 2026;149:422–31. https://doi.org/10.1093/brain/awaf3987.

Willis WD, Westlund KN. Neuroanatomy of the pain system and of the pathways that modulate pain. J Clin Neurophysiol. 1997;14(1):2–31. https://doi.org/10.1097/00004691-1997010000-00002.

Woolf CJ. Evidence for a central component of post-injury pain hypersenitivity. Nature. 1983;306(5944):686–8. https://doi.org/10.1038/306686a0.

Zeiglgänsberger W. Substance P and pain chronicity. Cell Tissue Res. 2019;375:227–41. https://doi.org/10.1007/s0441-018-2922-y.

Errors in Language and Logic Call for Epistemic Discipline

Abstract A prominent theme in this Handbook is the correct usage of language and of logic, as effectiveness in academic and clinical communication depends upon agreement on what words and concepts denote and on the consequent ability to argue logically and validly.

Already, certain topics regarding misnomers (errors in language) and fallacies (errors in reasoning) have been identified. These include pain being conceptualised as a thing with agentive properties, conflation between nociception and pain, confusion between stimulus and response and failure to distinguish the perspective of the pain observer from that of the pain experiencer.

This chapter presents a deeper dissection, from an epistemological point of view, of these and other misnomers and fallacies in the pain medicine literature. These arguments are extended to constructs that are shown to be based more on speculation than on fact. Approaches to remediating misnomers, improving the quality of argument and to critically appraising constructs are offered.

Epistemic discipline in the use of language and logic seems necessary and desirable both towards advancing understanding of the *aporia* of pain and to developing logical consistency in the field of pain medicine, as a prelude to improving the quality of patient care.

> Falsehood flies, and truth comes limping after it, so that when men become undeceived, it is too late …
>
> (Jonathan Swift, The Examiner No.14, Thursday 9/11/1710)

> A main source of our failure to understand is that we do not command a clear view of the use of our words.
>
> (Ludwig Wittgenstein 1953, #122 Philosophical Investigations)

> Logical errors are, I think, of greater practical importance than many people believe; they enable their perpetrators to hold the comfortable opinion on every subject in turn. (Bertrand Russell 1945:93)

> By exposing the counterfeits of reason, we can better recognize and value good reasoning which is conducive to better living for individuals and society at large. (Douglas Groothius 2023:75)

M. Cohen, J. Quintner, *A Philosophical Handbook for Pain Medicine Practice*,
https://doi.org/10.1007/978-981-92-1682-6_8

The science of nociception, the study of pain and pain medicine as a clinical discipline have together introduced a new vocabulary to define and describe concepts that have revolutionised this area of knowledge over the last half-century (Cohen et al. 2022). As in other fields of medicine, precision in terminology is necessary for effective communication between clinicians (Yagin and de Fernandes 2024) and between clinicians and patients (Henry and Matthias 2018; Cosic et al. 2019) to ensure patient safety and promote therapeutic effectiveness. This is particularly so in today's world where scientific and technological developments are rapidly occurring and many new terms enter language. To avoid confusion, standardisation of the meaning and usage of common terms is of fundamental importance.

Much of the terminology currently used in pain medicine has been drawn from various specialised fields, including but not limited to neurophysiology, neuroscience, psychology and psychiatry. However, problems have arisen when their denotation and connotation in the original discipline were not clear, which increases the potential for inaccurate or misleading usage when the terms are applied in the context of pain science and medicine. Physicians can perpetuate this problem by giving "diagnoses of exclusion" or using poor explanations, oversimplifications, conflicting diagnostic criteria or vague historical terms that have evolved into something else (Cohen et al. 2013).

Words are the currency of argument. Just as it is important to identify imprecise use of language, so is it equally necessary to recognise faulty reasoning that may render argument invalid. Attention to both is required to maintain epistemic discipline, defined here as a critical approach to evaluating information before accepting it as knowledge.

Errors in Language (Misnomers)

A misnomer is a name or a term that is incorrectly, improperly or misleadingly applied. Misnomers may be terms that were coined before the true nature of the object or phenomenon under discussion was understood. When these misunderstandings become linked to the object or phenomenon, they can become accepted knowledge and spread widely within the medical community (Manikat and Chopra 2023).

For example, the popular nineteenth-century condition neurasthenia ("weakness of the nerves") was based upon the concept of a physiological depletion of the body's finite reserves of electrical "nerve force" (Beard 1881). In this case, the misnomer was not necessarily incorrect because, at the time of its creation, it conveyed accepted knowledge.

Painful Stimulus

In biology, a stimulus is an object, event or factor capable of inciting a physiological response. Use of the term "painful stimulus", which permeates the literature, commits two fundamental errors. The first is to confuse stimulus and response. In this context, it is the response—the experience labelled "pain"—that is "painful". A stimulus that might ultimately induce pain is not in and of itself "painful". Following from the IASP ontology of pain terms (IASP 1979), the only correct adjective to describe a stimulus here is "noxious". The second error is to conceptualise the pain experience as a "thing"—an inanimate, material object—that has causal agency. By contrast, the pain experience can also be conceptualised as a process that may have agency, but this is not usual usage.[1]

Similarly, "nociceptive stimulus" remains in the taxonomy, defined as "an actually or potentially tissue damaging event transduced and encoded by nociceptors". The first objection is that this hardly differs at all from "a stimulus that is damaging or threatens damage to normal tissues", which is the definition of a noxious stimulus, one that is capable of activating nociceptors. The second objection is the paradoxical use of the suffix "-ceptive", which is clearly a property of a receptor but here is tied to a stimulus. This leads to the circular argument that a nociceptive stimulus is one that activates nociceptors. But that is what a noxious stimulus does. A stimulus that may induce pain is neither "painful" nor "nociceptive"; by definition, such a stimulus is "noxious".

Pain Fibres/Pathway/System

"Pain nerves", "pain fibres" and "pain pathways" are all misnomers, as they imply the erroneous notion that pain itself is a message—a "thing"—transmitted by neural mechanisms from an origin to the brain. Nerve fibres and pathways are indeed required to electrically encode and transmit information following nociception. However, that information refers to a noxious stimulus and is not "pain", which is a whole-organism experience. The only correct terms for this neural substrate are "nociceptive fibres" and "nociceptive pathways".

The concept of a "system" is of "a regularly interacting or interdependent group of items forming a unified whole" (Merriam-Webster). Does this system concept apply to "pain", as it may apply to the visual or auditory systems? In these latter two cases, the distinction is made between a stimulus, an apparatus adequate to detect that stimulus and the response to that stimulus. Each of those systems is labelled by its response (visual or auditory) rather than by its stimulus (photic or phonic). However, "pain" is a more complex and non-linear experience than sight or hearing, especially in verbal humans. Is the nexus between a noxious stimulus and pain sufficiently analogous to the coupling of a photic stimulus and vision or a phonic stimulus and hearing to be conceptualised as a "system"? If so, then the appropriate adjective should be "noxious" but the concept of a "noxious system" is unlikely to be acceptable. "Nociceptive" could be used but would then contrast to those other

---

[1] See also chapter "Trying to Gain Traction on a Slippery Subject".

sensory systems by being labelled by reference to its stimulus rather than its response.

This argument is summarised here:

Stimulus	Apparatus to detect and process stimulus	Response	Lay term (English)	"System"
Photic	Visual	Vision	Seeing	Visual
Phonic	Auditory	Audition	Hearing	Auditory
Noxious	Nociceptive	Pain	Pain	?Nociceptive

Taken together, these considerations suggest that the concept of a "pain system" is of limited utility.

Pain Sensitivity/Insensitivity/Hypersensitivity

The concept of "pain sensitivity" appears to make sense because its connotation is the ability to tolerate pain, as in, "it takes a lot of stimulus for me to acknowledge that I am hurting". This is often incorrectly asserted as "I have a high threshold for pain", when clearly that "threshold" has been surpassed. "Pain sensitivity" is shorthand for "sensitivity to pain", the basic premise of which is that pain is a stimulus, reflecting the fundamental error of considering pain to be a "thing". The pain experience is a response; "being sensitive" is itself a response. It follows that an organism cannot be "sensitive" to its own response.

The psychophysical concept of "pain sensitivity" originated in the mid-twentieth century, defined by Hardy et al. (1940) as the level of *experimental* stimulation that produces a "painful response" (or, more correctly, a response that is a pain experience). That can be rewritten as the level of intensity of a noxious stimulus that induces a pain experience. This was used synonymously with the concept of a "threshold" for a response of "pain" (or the "pain threshold"—see below). But *threshold* is a property of a stimulus, not of a response. These researchers used the term "pain sensibility" to describe the intensity of pain experienced in response to suprathreshold stimuli. This experience terminates at "pain tolerance" when the subject says "I cannot take any more stimulus". In contrast to "pain sensitivity", "pain sensibility" is a property of the response, not of the stimulus.

"Pain sensitivity" and "pain sensibility" have become confused in the peer-reviewed pain literature. Both terms perpetuate the notion that pain is a "thing" to which one might be "sensitive" or "sensible".

As corollaries, the terms "pain insensitivity" and "pain hypersensitivity" reflect the same fundamental error. "Pain insensitivity" is a term that was historically assigned to a group of conditions known as "congenital insensitivity to pain". However, this explicitly portrays pain as a "thing", thus conflating pain and nociception (Weisman et al. 2021). These authors suggest that "congenital nociceptor deficiency" is the only accurate term to describe this group of conditions (Weisman et al. 2019). "Pain hypersensitivity" can be traced to Woolf's pioneering report of injury-induced increases in the excitability of the decerebrate rat's flexion reflex (Woolf 1983), a phenomenon thought to arise in part from changes in activity in the spinal cord. Woolf suggested that those changes following tissue injury in the rat "parallel the sensory disturbances found in man", which he referred to as "pain hypersensitivity". However, an increase in objective excitability of a reflex does not allow any valid inference concerning subjective "sensory disturbances" in humans.

Pain is not a material "thing" to which an organism might be sensitive or insensitive or hypersensitive. It follows that this particular notion of pain as a causative agent is untenable. "Pain sensitivity" and related terms should be abandoned.

Pain Threshold

The IASP defines pain threshold as the minimum intensity of a stimulus perceived as painful by a subject (or leads to inferred pain behaviour in non-verbal beings) (Merskey and Bogduk 1994). This definition is unfortunate, as it perpetuates the misnomer of the "painful stimulus". So, to what does "threshold" actually refer? Is it a quality of the stimulus—its "noxiousness"—or a quality of the response—the propensity of a respondent to experience pain? The latter is especially pertinent, as a person might respond as much to an innocuous stimulus as to an actually noxious one.

Furthermore, the term has become a source both of pride—"I have a high pain threshold"—and of stigmatisation—"they have a low pain threshold"—when clearly what is being referred to here is the person's ability to *tolerate* the experience. Such contamination should not be allowed in a formal discipline, such that the term "pain threshold" should be discarded in scientific parlance in favour of "pain-inducing stimulus intensity" as a general term, with more specific terms referring to the type of stimulus used, such as mechanical, thermal or chemical.

Spatial Summation of Pain

Summation describes the act or process of adding things together. The term was introduced to the psychophysical literature by Hardy and Oppel (1937) as the "spatial summation of the end organ responses" in a study of sensitivity (as a response) to non-penetrating infra-red radiation applied to various skin sites. These authors postulated that the sensation experienced in response to this radiation was a function of the intensity of the stimulus and an "ability to add the separate effects of end organs in widely distributed areas". Clearly, these comments applied only to criteria for the stimulus to be registered by the "end-organ".

Somehow this concept was transmuted into "spatial summation of pain" by Hardy et al. (1940). This term, which has prevailed in the literature since then (Defrin et al. 2003; Lautenbacher et al. 2001; Raz et al. 2015), refers not to any stimulus but rather to the response, namely pain. For example, Price et al. (1978) referred to "prolonged summation of heat-induced second pain". It is clear that "spatial summation of pain" is a misnomer, as it refers to electrophysiological events that might "summate" to induce activation of nociceptors but not a pain experience. This is another example of conflation between nociception and pain. A correct term for this phenomenon would be spatial summation of stimuli to engage nociception.

Pain Processing

Processing refers to a series of actions. "Pain processing" stems from the proposition that pain is a "signal"—that is, a thing with agentive properties—that can be manipulated by the nervous system. This proposition flies in the face of the fact that a pain experience is always the final outcome of complex neurophysiological and psychological mechanisms (Melzack 1961). As this experience itself is a final outcome, it cannot be "processed" further.

As an example of this misnomer, a study's findings were said to be consistent with the hypothesis that "stimulus expectancy effects on pain may involve systems working in concert to alter pain processing both downstream at the level of the dorsal horn and upstream at the level of S1" (Henderson et al. 2020:9). What is being "processed" is information from activated nociceptors. The correct term should be "processing of noxious information" or, as a shorthand, "nociceptive processing". But the relationship between that neurophysiological process and the pain experience itself is elusive. It is not "pain" that is being "processed".

The same criticism can be applied to a therapeutic approach known as Pain Reprocessing Therapy (Ashar et al. 2022, 2025). It follows from the above that "reprocessing" of pain is both logically and biologically untenable. The pain experience may well be modulated by "psychological" factors but there are no grounds to infer that it can occur independently of engagement of nociception in some form (Cohen et al. 2022; Weisman et al. 2026).

Pain Amplification

The term "symptom amplification" was initially used to describe increased bodily sensations in psychologically distressed patients (Barsky 1979). The concept was then applied to nociceptive signalling (Woolf 1983) and to central sensitisation of nociception (Woolf 2018). That leaves "pain amplification" with an ambiguous connotation, caught between a form of "nociceptive processing" and a psychological phenomenon. Because of this confusing ambiguity, taken together with "amplification" being a form of "processing", the term is best avoided.

Pain Chronification

"Pain chronification" is said to refer to a process whereby a temporary pain experience becomes persistent. This has been attributed to "... an imbalance between pain amplification and pain inhibition; genetic, environmental, and biopsychosocial factors determine the risk, the degree, and time-course of chronification" (Morlion et al. 2018:1169). This concept is another example of conflating a pseudo-definition—"chronification" means "changing from temporary to persistent"—with a speculative mechanism—"imbalance between pain amplification and pain inhibition"—and causative factors—"genetic, environmental and biopsychosocial". Such a speculation that embraces all possibilities does not advance understanding. The term "pain chronification" should be defined strictly as denoting a pain experience changing from temporary to persistent or it should be abandoned. In all of these examples, it would seem that ultimately pain is being held responsible for its own modulation, which is an example of the logical fallacy of circular reasoning. The fundamental epistemological error, again, is to consider pain as a "thing".

Conditioned Pain Modulation

There is a phenomenon in which the deliberate application of a novel stimulus appears to decrease an existing pain experience. In the experimental animal literature, this effect has been attributed to a specific lower brainstem-mediated mechanism that inhibits transmission of nociceptive information, termed "diffuse noxious inhibitory control (DNIC)" (Yarnitsky 2010).

In humans, this experimental phenomenon has been transmuted into the construct of conditioned pain modulation (CPM), described as "psychophysical paradigms in which a conditioning stimulus is used to affect a test stimulus" (Woolf 2018). Here, the "test stimulus" is a "painful stimulus", the response to which is modified by prior application of a "conditioning stimulus" (Yarnitsky 2010; Yarnitsky et al. 2010). In fact the "conditioning" stimulus is itself not only noxious but also more intense than the "test" one. This has led to the extraordinary conceptualisation of this phenomenon as "pain inhibits pain" that may well have inspired the unwarranted application of "treatments" for pain that themselves induce pain (Weisman et al. 2021).

There are three major problems here, not so much with the phenomenon itself as with the nomenclature and inference regarding mechanism. Firstly, the term "painful stimulus" is an unacceptable misnomer: noxious stimulus is the appropriate term. Secondly, the choice of the term "conditioned pain modulation" is unfortunate, as it resembles but is by no means the same as the "conditioned" stimulus used in behavioural psychology. Thirdly, what in fact is being "conditioned"? If there is an implicit presumption that DNIC is the underlying mechanism, then it is not pain that is being "modulated" but rather the processing of noxious information.

The construct of CPM needs to be reformulated, initially by using correct terminology and then revisiting the psychophysical phenomena it purports to describe. In the meantime, reverting to the older term "counter-irritation analgesia" would resolve the identified problems. As Gammon and Starr (1941) concluded, having used themselves as subjects: "Irrespective of the type of pain and counterirritant, a definite pattern usually appeared: the application of counter-irritation caused temporary relief; its removal was also followed by temporary relief" (p. 20) (Table 1).

Table 1 Summary of common misnomers in pain medicine and suggested remediation. (Modified from Cohen et al. 2022)

Misnomer	Problem	Recommendation
Pain sensitivity (Pain insensitivity Pain hypersensitivity)	Undefined in IASP lexicon Pain not a material "thing" to which one is sensitive	Discard
Pain threshold	Ambiguous usage IASP definition: The minimum intensity of a stimulus that is perceived as painful. More correctly: The minimum intensity of a stimulus that induces a pain experience.	Replace with: Pain-inducing stimulus intensity (PISI), specifying whether the stimulus is – mechanical (touch, pressure, movement) – thermal (heat, cold) – chemical (extrinsic, ischaemia)
Pain fibres/pathways/system	Undefined in IASP lexicon Nerves do not transmit "pain"	Replace with: nociceptive fibres/pathways/system
Pain processing	Undefined in IASP lexicon Pain is not a material "thing" that is "processed"	Replace with: nociceptive processing, or processing of noxious/nociceptive information
Pain amplification	Undefined in IASP lexicon Ambiguous	Discard
Chronification of pain	Undefined in IASP lexicon Arbitrary	Discard
Painful stimulus	IASP defines *nociceptive stimulus* as: An actually or potentially tissue-damaging event transduced and encoded by nociceptors.	Replace with: noxious stimulus
Spatial summation of pain	Undefined in IASP lexicon Conflation of nociception and pain	Replace with: spatial summation of nociception (SSN)
Conditioned pain modulation	Undefined in IASP lexicon Not pain that is being "modulated" but rather processing of noxious information	"Counter-irritation analgesia", pending psychophysical and linguistic reappraisal

Errors in Reasoning

Misnomers are mistakes with respect to the meaning and usage of words and should not be confused with fallacies, which are examples of faulty reasoning that render an argument invalid. In a formal fallacy or *non-sequitur*, a conclusion does not follow validly from its premises, whereas in an informal fallacy, the error may be found in the content of the premises, even if the logical structure is valid. However, fallacies are incorrect no matter how they appear. In this way, unsubstantiated assertions may be presented as if they were facts (McMullin 2000).

Reification: Pain Being Conceptualised as a "Thing"

The concept that pain, which is an experience, is not only a concrete entity (or "thing") but also an agent that can be held responsible for neurophysiological changes is an example of the fallacy of presumption known as "reification" (Arp et al. 2018). This term is derived from the Latin *res* ("thing") and *facere* ("to make"). Another name for "reification" is the "fallacy of misplaced concreteness" (Whitehead and Sherburne 1929). A common instance of this fallacy is "Pain can produce increased muscle contraction, tone, or trigger points" (Chimenti et al. 2018). The assertion that pain is a "thing" that can be "reprocessed" by the person's brain (Ashar et al. 2022) is another instance of reification.

The error is to presume that an abstract entity can be taken as having material, physical existence. This is not to argue against abstract reasoning, which plays a fundamental role in science. However, as pointed out in the examples above, fallacious reasoning can lead to inaccurate scientific explanations of abstract phenomena. This error—that pain is a material causative agent—frequently occurs in the pain literature and is compounded by the consequent circular argument that pain can be its own cause.

Mereological Fallacy

According to some authors, the brain produces pain when it perceives that danger to body tissue exists and that action is required (Butler and Moseley 2013). This leads to the proposition, "As part of the brain weighs the world, it makes a value judgment on the inputs and responds … when you are in danger, the brain calls upon many systems to get you out of trouble" (Butler and Moseley 2013:42).

This proposal is reminiscent of the "Cartesian theatre" depicted by philosopher Daniel Dennett (1993), in which a range of possible choices for action are presented to a homunculus ("little man") residing in the brain, who can then instantaneously decide on the most appropriate course of action and instruct the relevant brain processes to proceed accordingly.

This approach conceptualises pain as an output of a brain that has "decided" that the person is in danger, even in contexts with no obvious evidence of such danger.

Such an approach is neuro-essentialist, which is a way of explaining human psychological experience (of which pain is an example) solely by reference to the brain and its activity (Schultz 2018). This is an example of the mereological fallacy, that is, "ascribing to parts attributes that can be ascribed intelligibly only to the wholes of which they are parts" (Bennett and Hacker 2008).

Although each of these assertions constitutes a logically consistent argument, they are nonetheless fallacious as the content of the premises is speculation rather than fact. The proposition that the brain "decides" when a person is in danger is untestable and therefore cannot be supported.

Teleological Explanation

Another aspect of this brain-centred approach is the assertion that pain is "a biopsychosocial phenomenon" with an adaptive, protective role (Moseley and Butler 2015:17). This approach claims to be a radical shift in the way pain is conceptualised, "from that of a marker of tissue damage or disease to that of the perceived need to protect body tissue" (Moseley and Butler 2015: 807). This reconceptualisation is based on neuromatrix theory, as formulated by Melzack (1990). When discussing phantom limb phenomena, Melzack claimed that "neural networks within the brain generate all the qualities of experience that are felt to originate in the body; inputs from the body may trigger or modulate the output of the networks but are *not essential for any of the qualities of the experience*" (p. 90; emphasis added here). In other words, no longer were "inputs from the body" necessary for the pain experience. According to Moseley (2007), this output is determined by an implicit perception of threat, not by the state of tissues or by any actual threat to them.

This conceptual shift has been quoted on numerous occasions, both in the peer-reviewed scientific literature (Beales et al. 2016; Moseley and Butler 2017; Leake et al. 2019; Ryan et al. 2024; Wand et al. 2023) and in social media.[2] It exemplifies the teleological fallacy, in which phenomena are explained in terms of the presumed purpose they serve or the ends they meet, rather than in terms of the cause by which they arise (Mayr 1992).

On what authority, let alone evidence, does a pain experience in and of itself serve a purpose? How does a brain "perceive" that there is a "need" to "protect"? From what is a pain experience protecting the organism? How does a pain experience do this? These questions have never been addressed by those responsible for such teleological assertions.[3]

---

[2] [Tame the Beast. It's Time to Rethink Persistent Pain, Available at https://www.tamethebeast.org/#tame-the-beast]; [Essential Pain Fact 1, Pain Revolution, Available at https://www.painrevolution.org/epf1; What is pain? Available at https://www.painaustralia.org.au/about-pain/painaustralia-what-is-pain].

[3] See chapter "Translation into the Clinic" for further discussion of "pain-as-a-protector".

Illusory Truth Effect

Repetition of a fallacious argument is an example of the "illusory truth effect", through which the more often information is encountered, the more truthful that information is considered to be (Dechêne et al. 2010). This effect holds true, even when information comes from sources of unknown validity (Barber and Hassan 2021). It has also been shown that repetition of misinformation can bias people's judgement of accuracy and, as a result, create a vicious circle in which it will be perceived as true and therefore more often and widely spread (Vellani et al. 2023). An example is the persistence of the joint assertions that a pain experience is learned and therefore can be unlearned (Cordier and Diers 2018), despite those assertions having been refuted (Shanks 2010).

Errors in Constructs

A similar approach of dissecting language and logic can be applied to distinguishing fact from conjecture contained in some constructs commonly used in Pain Medicine.

Pain Catastrophising

The term "catastrophising" means "to view or present a situation as considerably worse than it actually is" (Macmillan Dictionary). It was coined by psychoanalyst Albert Ellis (1962) to describe a person's preoccupation with anticipated disasters. By 1990, catastrophising had entered the pain literature in two forms, as "an explanatory construct for variations in pain and depression in chronic pain patients" and as "a maladaptive coping strategy that intensifies the experience of pain and depression" (Sullivan and D'Eon 1990:260). However, after examining the instruments used to identify these constructs, these authors found that catastrophising was of limited use in explaining such variation, which was more likely to reflect "the cognitive and affective components of dysphoria".

By 1998, the definition had become "an exaggerated negative orientation toward pain stimuli (*sic*) and pain experience" (Sullivan et al. 1998). However, Turner and Aaron (2001) were unsure whether pain-related catastrophising referred to a stable personality disposition (a trait) or a situational response (a state). In yet another modification, catastrophising became "an exaggerated negative mental set brought to bear during actual or anticipated painful experiences". Nevertheless, it was unclear whether this "mental set" referred to "an appraisal, a coping strategy or a maladaptive belief" (Quartana et al. 2009:13).

It has been stated that "pain catastrophising is an important psychological factor that influences pain response (*sic*) and disability, but paradoxically no conceptual agreement is available at present that can explain what catastrophising really is" (Petrini and Arendt-Nielsen 2020:12). This review goes on to assert that pain catastrophising "is an emotional regulator strategy, a catastrophic worry, constituting an interplay between a ruminative process and personality trait characteristics related to the BIS[4]" (Petrini and Arendt-Nielsen 2020:12). Here "catastrophic worry" is conceptualised as an "emotional... strategy", then linked to a hypothetical mechanism. The apparent conclusion is that people who are prone to "pain catastrophising"—those for whom "pain vulnerability" is a "risk—are likely to have a "complex interplay of biological and psychosocial factors".

In overview, not only has the concept of "pain catastrophising" never been defined clearly but also it has been confused and conflated in the literature. Proposals vary from "an exaggerated negative cognitive-affective orientation toward pain" (Schütze et al. 2018) to "a set of maladaptive beliefs concerning actual or anticipated pain experiences that induce pain-related fear responses which in turn foster disability" (Conti et al. 2020) and to "a set of exaggerated and negative cognitive-emotional responses to actual or anticipated painful sensations, leading individuals to magnify or exaggerate the threat of pain stimuli and to feel helpless" (Varallo et al. 2021).

However, pain is already defined as "an unpleasant sensory and emotional experience" (IASP 1979; Raja et al. 2020). Who is to judge the appropriateness of such an experience? The questions left unanswered are whether "catastrophising" is part of the pain experience or is it a reflection on the experience, and is its purpose to serve the experiencer or the observer? Perhaps "catastrophising" is best avoided and replaced with suffering or existential distress that may accompany the pain experience.

Fear Avoidance and Kinesiophobia

Fear Avoidance

The fear-avoidance model was proposed to explain one aspect of the behavioural dimension of the pain experience, namely the avoidance of movements or activities based on the fear of increased pain or reinjury (Spisak et al. 2020). According to this model, to confront the experience by viewing pain as a temporary nuisance and to be motivated to resume social and leisure activities is said to be adaptive behaviour. By contrast, to avoid activities that could occasion further experience of pain is said to be non-adaptive, hence "fear-avoidant" behaviour. That in itself is a strange label, as the behaviour is more likely to be "pain-avoidant", which in turn raises the

[4] "behavioural inhibition system".

question of distinguishing that from "injury-avoidant", while at the same time possibly meaning avoidance of fear.

The proponents argue that such a response is "likely to be exaggerated pain perception *(sic),* involving a marked desynchrony between pain sensation, on the one hand, and pain experience and pain behaviour on the other" (Slade et al. 1983:405). But what is this "desynchrony" between the sensory and behavioural aspects of the pain experience? This argument omits the cognitive aspect, which together with the sensory aspect would determine the "pain behaviour". Indeed, does "exaggerated pain perception" actually mean an "exaggerated perception of pain", which would imply that pain is a "thing" that is perceived, or does it refer to the cognitive dimension of the pain experience, in contrast to the sensory dimension? If a person's cognitive appraisal is that an activity is associated with an increase in their pain experience, why is that necessarily "exaggerated" let alone "maladaptive"? Yet, it is claimed without evidence that "[F]ear and anxiety [that] leads to avoidance of activities, expectations about increased pain, and more self-reported disability" (Karlsson et al. 2016:2).

Dissection of the construct of "fear avoidance" reveals that its fundamental tenet, "exaggerated pain perception", is a judgement of the observer and not of the experiencer. By also claiming that this behaviour is "non-adaptive", the construct is simultaneously teleological—pain behaviour is purposed towards healing or recovery—and moralistic—pain behaviour should be "adaptive".

Kinesiophobia

Kinesiophobia ("fear of movement") is a construct parallel with fear avoidance, described as "an excessive, irrational, and debilitating fear of physical movement and activity resulting from a feeling of vulnerability to painful injury or reinjury" (Kori and Miller 1990). Again, this is a judgement of the observer, that the behaviour of the experiencer arises out of trait "vulnerability" and generates a "phobia", which by definition is an irrational fear, that in turn is "excessive and debilitating". How can an observer judge that a pain experience being worsened by movement is not only "irrational" but also a reflection of "vulnerability"? Indeed, the TAMPA Scale for assessing kinesiophobia (Miller et al. 1991) contains questions to which the answers given may be rational and entirely appropriate to the situation faced by the respondent (Lundberg et al. 2009).

There is no real conceptual difference between these two constructs that seek to ascribe observed behaviour to fear, whether of movement, of pain or of reinjury. In one (fear-avoidance), a person's fear of reinjury following physical activity is attributed to the possibility that the person had made an incorrect assumption (Vlaeyen et al. 1995). In the other (kinesiophobia), the role of current pain intensity, underlying organic pathology or nociception is thought to play no part (Vlaeyen et al. 1995). Which of these is the "incorrect assumption"? Both are challenged by the phenomenon of nociplastic pain (Kosek et al. 2016), which invokes the possibility of altered central nociceptive function being responsible for pain.[5] Perhaps, then, in the case of nociplastic pain, the cognitive appraisal that physical activity increases the experience of pain is neither irrational nor excessive nor based on fear.

None of this is to deny the importance and challenge of interpreting the behaviour of a person experiencing pain. Perhaps heuristics based on exploring the individual's cognitive appraisal of their own predicament in their own words rather than through instruments such as these may be more valid and effective.

Maladaptive Pain

This term reflects a common teleological argument that pain is an "alarm system" preserved through evolution for a specific function (Butler and Moseley 2013:19; Walters 2019). According to this argument, the "alarm" function of pain can malfunction. As Dickinson et al. (2010) assert, "maladaptive pain may occur in the absence of ongoing noxious stimuli and does not promote health and repair" (p. 1636). Apart from the unanswered question as to how it is possible for a pain experience *per se* to "promote health and repair", it is now understood that nociplastic pain (Kosek et al. 2016) and "chronic pain" (ICD-11) (Nicholas et al. 2019) may "occur in the absence of ongoing noxious stimuli".

The perspective of "maladaptive pain", also known as maldynia (Dickinson et al. 2010), has been traced to misconceptions surrounding the group of conditions known as "congenital insensitivity to pain", itself a misnomer. This argument fails when critically examined, as it stems from conflation of pain experience and nociception (Weisman et al. 2019). "Maladaptive" pain goes even further, adducing a moral dimension of how a person experiencing pain should feel (Quintner et al. 2011).

Why Does Epistemic Discipline Matter?

The examples of misnomers, faulty reasoning and flawed constructs presented here call for more epistemic discipline in pain science and pain medicine. Misnomers can be corrected by consensus and logical errors can be addressed once identified. Dissecting constructs is more difficult. The use of heuristic methods towards discovery or problem-solving is necessary and desirable. It is also necessary that heuristic tools such as constructs distinguish between agreed fact and speculation (Weisman et al. 2020). Conjectures are not facts until they have survived rigorous attempts at refutation. This requires attention to both the accuracy of the premises in an argument and the validity of the argument itself.

[5] See chapter "The Salient Role of Nociception".

For example, a general proposition in the form of *There exists a psychological factor that we cannot define but which plays a role in the pain experience of individuals who are prone to it* may appear valid, until its teleological and tautological traps are recognised. This is not to deny the potential heuristic value of models; for example, "fear-avoidance" may appear plausible but as its purported mechanisms are not testable, as shown above, it does not survive scrutiny.

In his Medawar lecture, the philosopher of science Peter Lipton (2005) wrote:

"To make a scientific claim is to assert that the claim is true". As he puts it, "... scientific inferences are often driven by asking how good an explanation a given hypothesis would provide of the phenomena if it were true, and then, *if it would be good enough, inferring that it is true*" (emphasis in original). In other words, "the activity of explanation itself supposes truth" (p. 39). This recalls the admonition from Medawar himself, that the evidence that leads to a conclusion cannot be then used to justify the veracity of that conclusion (Medawar 1969). Just because the conjecture appears plausible does not mean it is true. A significant problem with failing to recognise content errors or logical fallacies in conjectures is that their propagation can give rise to the illusory truth effect.

In everyday life, minor levels of inconsistent use of language and invalid logical arguments are tolerated and accommodated. However, in scientific and medical communication, agreed terminologies along with sound and consistent arguments are essential for generating valid knowledge and translating that into the clinic. The importance of these considerations is not limited to the clinical and academic arenas but also has major implications for people living with pain that adversely affects their quality of life. One of the more powerful therapeutic tools available to the clinical pain practitioner, irrespective of their background discipline, is to present a clear, honest and epistemologically sound explanation of the predicament of those who seek their help (Cohen et al. 2022).

References

Arp R, Barbone S, Bruce M. Bad arguments: 100 of the most important fallacies in Western philosophy. Hoboken: Wiley; 2018. p. 378–81.

Ashar YK, Gordon R, Schubiner H, et al. Effect of pain reprocessing therapy vs placebo and usual care for patients with chronic back pain: a randomised controlled trial. JAMA Psychiatry. 2022;790(1):13–23. https://doi.org/10.1001/jamapsychiatry.2021.2669.

Ashar YK, Low EL, Knight K, Schubiner H, Gordon A, LeRoux A, Lumley MA, Wager TD. Pain reprocessing therapy vs placebo and usual care for patients with chronic back pain: 5-year follow-up of a randomized clinical trial. JAMA Psychiatry. 2025;82(10):1049–51. https://doi.org/10.1001/jamapsychiatry.2025.1844.

Barber SJ, Hassan A. The effects of repetition frequency on the illusory truth effect. Cogn Res. 2021;6:38. https://doi.org/10.1186/s41325-021-00301-5.

Barsky AJ. Patients who amplify bodily sensations. Ann Intern Med. 1979;91:63–70. https://doi.org/10.7326/0003-4819-91-1-63.

Beales D, Fried K, Nicholas M, Blyth F, Finniss D, Moseley GL. Management of musculoskeletal pain in a compensable environment: implementation of helpful and unhelpful models of care in

supporting recovery and return to work. Best Pract Clin Rheumatol. 2016;30:445–67. https://doi.org/10.1016/j.berh.2016.08.011.
Beard GM. American nervousness, its causes and consequences: a supplement to nervous exhaustion (neurasthenia). New York NY: Putnam; 1881. p. 1–17.
Bennett MR, Hacker PMS. History of cognitive neuroscience. Chichester: Wiley; 2008. p. 68–103.
Butler DS, Moseley GL. Explain Pain. 2nd ed. Adelaide: Noigroup Publications; 2013.
Chimenti RL, Frey-Law LA, Sluka KA. A mechanism-based approach to physical therapist management of pain. Phys Ther. 2018;98(5):302–14. https://doi.org/10.1093/ptj/pzy030.
Cohen HKS, Luther A, Hart CA. Confusing medical terms: disease that may or may not exist. Q J Med. 2013;106(7):617–21. https://doi.org/10.1093/qjmed/hct076.
Cohen M, Weisman A, Quintner J. Pain is not a "thing": how that error affects language and logic in pain medicine. J Pain. 2022;23:1283–93. https://doi.org/10.1016/j.jpain.2022.03.235.
Conti Y, Vatine JJ, Levy S, Levin Meltz Y, Hamdan S, Elkana O. Pain catastrophizing mediates the association between mindfulness and psychological distress in chronic pain syndrome. Pain Pract. 2020;20:714–23. https://doi.org/10.1111/papr.12899.
Cordier L, Diers M. Learning and unlearning of pain. Biomedicines 2018;6:67. https://doi.org/10.3390/biomedicines6020067.
Cosic F, Kimmel L, Edwards E. Patient comprehension of common orthopedic terminology. Health Lit Res Pract. 2019;3(3):e187–93. https://doi.org/10.3928/24748307-20190624-04.
Dechêne A, Stahl C, Hansen J, Wänke M. The truth about the truth: a meta-analytic review of the truth effect. Personal Soc Psychol Rev. 2010;14:238–57. https://doi.org/10.1177/1088868309352251.
Defrin R, Ronat A, Ravid A, Peretz C. Spatial summation of pressure pain: effect of body region. Pain. 2003;106:471–80. https://doi.org/10.1016/j.pain.2003.09.010.
Dennett DC. Consciousness explained. London: Penguin UK; 1993. p. 253–82.
Dickinson BD, Head CA, Gitlow S, Osbahr AJ III. Maldynia: pathophysiology and management of neuropathic and maladaptive pain—a report of the AMA Council on science and public health. Pain Med. 2010;11:1635–53. https://doi.org/10.1111/j.1526-4637.2010.00986.x.
Ellis A. Reason and emotion in psychotherapy. New York: Lyle Stuart; 1962. p. 71.
Gammon GD, Starr I. Studies on the relief of pain by counterirritation. J Clin Invest. 1941;20:13–20.
Groothuis D. Avoiding pitfalls in reasoning. Think. 2023;22(64):71–5. https://doi.org/10.1017/S1477175623000131.
Hardy J, Oppel T. Studies in temperature sensation. III. The sensitivity of the body to heat and the spatial summation of the end organ responses. J Clin Invest. 1937;16:533–40.
Hardy JD, Wolff HG, Goodell H, Studies on pain. A new method for measuring pain threshold: observations on spatial summation of pain. J Clin Invest. 1940;19:649–57.
Henderson LA, Di Pietro F, Youssef AM, Lee S, Tam S, Akhter R, Mills EP, Murray GM, Peck CC, Macey PM. Effect of expectation on pain processing: a psychophysics and functional MRI analysis. Front Neurosci. 2020;14:6. https://doi.org/10.3389/fnins.2020.00006.
Henry SG, Matthias MS. Patient-clinician communication about pain: a conceptual model and narrative review. Pain Med. 2018;19(11):2154–65. https://doi.org/10.1093/pm/pny003.
IASP. Pain terms: a list with definitions and notes on usage. Recommended by the IASP Subcommittee on taxonomy. Pain. 1979;6:247–52.
Karlsson L, Gerdle B, Takala E-P, Andersson G, Larsson B. Associations between psychological factors and the effect of home-based physical exercise in women with chronic neck and shoulder pain. SAGE Open Med. 2016;4:2050312116668933.
Kori S, Miller R. Kinesophobia: a new view of chronic pain behavior. Pain Manage. 1990;3:35–43.
Kosek E, Cohen M, Baron R, Gebhart GF, Mico J-A, Rice AS, Rief W, Sluka KA. Do we need a third mechanistic descriptor for chronic pain states? Pain. 2016;157:1382–6. https://doi.org/10.1097/j.pain.0000000000000507.
Lautenbacher JN, Nielsen J, Andersen T, Arendt-Nielsen L. Spatial summation of heat pain in males and females. Somatosens Mot Res. 2001;18:101–5. https://doi.org/10.1080/135578501012006192-1.

Leake HB, Heathcote LC, Simons LE, Stinson J, Kamper SJ, Williams CM, et al. Talking to teens about pain: a modified Delphi study of adolescent pain science education. Can J Pain. 2019;3(1):200–8. https://doi.org/10.1080/24740527.2019.1682934.
Lipton P. The Medawar lecture 2004: the truth about science. Philos Trans R Soc Lond Ser B Biol Sci. 2005;360:1259–69. https://doi.org/10.1098/rstb.2005.1660.
Lundberg M, Styf J, Jansson B. On what patients does the Tampa Scale for Kinesiophobia fit? Physiother Theory Pract. 2009;25:495–506. https://doi.org/10.3109/09593980802662160.
Macmillan Dictionary. "catastrophize". Available at: https://www.macmillandictionary.com/dictionary/british/catastrophize. Accessed 05 June 2025.
Manikat R, Chopra S. Medical misnomers are murky: time to memorialize and rename. Am J Med. 2023;136(12):1160–4. https://doi.org/10.1016/j.amjmed.2022.08.021.
Mayr E. The idea of teleology. J Hist Ideas. 1992;53(1):117–35.
McMullin RE. The new handbook of cognitive therapy techniques. New York: WW Norton and Company; 2000. p. 159–207.
Medawar PB. Induction and intuition in scientific thought. Oxford: Routledge; 1969.
Melzack R. The perception of pain. Sci Am. 1961;204(2):41–9.
Melzack R. Phantom limbs and the concept of a neuromatrix. Trends Neurosci. 1990;13:88–92. https://doi.org/10.1016/0166-2236(90)90179-e.
Merriam-Webster Dictionary. "system". Available at: https://www.merriamwebster.com/dictionary/system. Accessed 1 June 2025
Merskey H, Bogduk N. Pain terms, a current list with definitions and notes on usage. In: Merskey H, Bogduk N, editors. Classification of chronic pain, second edition, IASP task force on taxonomy. Seattle: IASP Press; 1994. p. 209–14.
Miller RP, Kori SH, Todd DD. The Tampa scale: a measure of kinesiophobia. Clin J Pain. 1991;7:51.
Morlion B, Coluzzi F, Aldington D, Kocot-Kepska M, Pergolizzi J, Mangas AC, Ahlbeck K, Kalso E. Pain chronification: what should a non-pain medicine specialist know? Curr Med Res Opin. 2018;34:1169–78. https://doi.org/10.1080/03007995.2018.1449738.
Moseley GL. Reconceptualising pain according to modern pain science. Phys Ther Rev. 2007;12:169–78. https://doi.org/10.1179/108331907X223010.
Moseley GL, Butler DS. Fifteen years of explaining pain: the past, present, and future. J Pain. 2015;16:807–13. https://doi.org/10.1016/j.jpain.2015.05.005.
Moseley GL, Butler DS. Explain pain supercharged. Adelaide: NOI Group; 2017.
Nicholas M, Vlaeyen JW, Rief W, Barke A, Aziz Q, Benoliel R, Cohen M, Evers S, Finnerup NB, First MB, Giamberidino MA, Kaasa S, Korwisi B, Kosek E, Lavand'homme P, Perrot S, Scholz J, Schug S, Svensson P, Vlaeyen JWS, Wang SJ. The IASP classification of chronic pain for ICD-11: chronic primary pain. Pain. 2019;160:28–37.
Petrini L, Arendt-Nielsen L. Understanding pain catastrophizing: putting pieces together. Front Psychol. 2020;11:1–18. https://doi.org/10.3389/fpsyg.2020.603420.
Price DD, Hayes RL, Ruda M, Dubner R. Spatial and temporal transformations of input to spinothalamic tract neurons and their relation to somatic sensations. J Neurophysiol. 1978;41:933–47. https://doi.org/10.1152/jn.1978.41.4.933.
Quartana PJ, Campbell CM, Edwards RR. Pain catastrophizing: a critical review. Expert Rev Neurother. 2009;9:745758. https://doi.org/10.1586/ern.09.34.
Quintner J, Buchanan D, Cohen M. Maldynia as a moral judgment? Pain Med. 2011;12:1130. https://doi.org/10.1111/j.1526-4637.2011.01174.x.
Raja SN, Carr DB, Cohen M, Finnerup NB, Flor H, Gibson S, Keefe F, Mogil JS, Ringkamp M, Sluka KA, Stevens B, Sullivan M, Tutelman P, Ushida T, Vader T. The revised IASP definition of pain: concepts, challenges, and compromise. Pain. 2020;161(9):1976–82. https://doi.org/10.1097/j.pain.0000000000001939.
Raz N, Granovsky Y, Defrin R. Investigating the neural processing of spatial summation of pain. The role of A-delta nociceptors. Exp Brain Res. 2015;233:405–13. https://doi.org/10.1007/s00221-014-4123-6.
Russell B. A history of Western philosophy. New York NY: Simon and Schuster; 1945.

Ryan CG, Karran EL, Wallwork SB, Pate JW, O'Keefe M, Fullen BM, et al. We are all in this together – whole of community pain science education campaign to promote better management of persistent pain. J Pain. 2024;25(4):902–17. https://doi.org/10.1016/j.jpain.2023.10.0254.
Schultz W. Neuroessentialism: theoretical and clinical considerations. J Humanist Psychol. 2018;58:607–39.
Schütze R, Rees C, Smith A, Slater H, Campbell JM, O'Sullivan P. How can we best reduce pain catastrophizing in adults with chronic noncancer pain? A systematic review and meta-analysis. J Pain. 2018;19:233–56. https://doi.org/10.1016/j.jpain.2017.09.010.
Shanks DR. Learning: from association to cognition. Annu Rev Psychol 2010;61:273–301. https://doi.org/10.1146/annurev.psych.093008.100519.
Slade PD, Troup JDG, Lethem J, Bentley G. The fear-avoidance model of exaggerated pain perception—I. Behav Res Ther. 1983;21:401–8.
Spisak T, Kincses B, Schlitt F, Zunhammer M, Schmidt-Wilcke T, Kincses ZT, Bingel U. Pain-free resting-state functional brain connectivity predicts individual pain sensitivity. Nat Commun. 2020;11:1–12. https://doi.org/10.1038/s41467-019-13785-z.
Sullivan MJ, D'Eon JL. Relation between catastrophizing and depression in chronic pain patients. J Abnorm Psychol. 1990;99:260–3. https://doi.org/10.1037/0021-843x.99.3.260.
Sullivan MJL, Stanish W, Waite H, Sullivan M, Tripp DA. Catastrophizing, pain, and disability in patients with soft tissue injuries. Pain. 1998;77:253–60. https://doi.org/10.1016/S0304-3959(98)00097-9.
Turner JA, Aaron LA. Pain-related catastrophizing: what is it? Clin J Pain. 2001;17:65–71. https://doi.org/10.1097/00002508-200103000-00009.
Varallo G, Giusti EM, Scarpina F, Cattivelli R, Capodaglio P, Castelnuovo G. The association of kinesiophobia and pain catastrophizing with pain-related disability and pain intensity in obesity and chronic lower-back pain. Brain Sci. 2021;11:11. https://doi.org/10.3390/brainsci11010011.
Vellani V, Zheng S, Ercelek D, Sharon T. The illusory truth effect leads to the spread of misinformation. Cognition. 2023;236:105421. https://doi.org/10.1016/j.cognition.2023.105421.
Vlaeyen JWS, Kole-Snijders AMJ, Boeren RGB, van Eek H. Fear of movement/(re)injury in chronic low back pain and its relation to behavioral performance. Pain. 1995;62:363–72. https://doi.org/10.1016/0304-3959(94)00279-N.
Walters ET. Adaptive mechanisms driving maladaptive pain: how chronic ongoing activity in primary nociceptors can enhance evolutionary fitness after severe injury. Philos Trans R Soc B. 2019;374:20190277. https://doi.org/10.1098/rstb.2019.0277.
Wand BM, Cashin AG, McAuley JH, Bagg MK, Orange GM, Moseley GL. The fit-for-purpose model: conceptualizing and managing chronic nonspecific low back pain as an information problem. Phys Ther. 2023;103(2):pzac151. https://doi.org/10.1093/ptj/pzac151.
Weisman A, Quintner J, Masharawi Y. Congenital insensitivity to pain: a misnomer. J Pain. 2019;20:1011–4. https://doi.org/10.1016/j.jpain.2019.01.331.
Weisman A, Quintner J, Galbraith M, Masharawi Y. Why are assumptions passed off as established knowledge? Med Hypotheses. 2020;140:109693. https://doi.org/10.1016/j.mehy.2020.109693.
Weisman A, Quintner J, Masharawi Y. Amplified pain syndrome – an insupportable assumption. JAMA Pediatr. 2021;17:557–8. https://doi.org/10.1001/jamapediatrics.2021.0111.
Weisman A, Quintner J, Cohen M. Adieu to an aphorism: nociception is necessary for pain. Brain. 2026;149:422–31. https://doi.org/10.1093/brain/awaf3987.
Whitehead AN, Sherburne DW. Process and reality. New York, NY: Macmillan; 1929. p. 11.
Wittgenstein L. Philosophical investigations. Anscombe GEM, Rhees R, editors. Anscombe GEM, translator. Oxford: Blackwell; 1953.
Woolf CJ. Evidence for a central component of post-injury pain hypersensitivity. Nature. 1983;306:686–8. https://doi.org/10.1038/306686a0.
Woolf CJ. Pain amplification - a perspective on the how, why, when, and where of central sensitization. J Appl Biobehav Res. 2018;23:e12124. https://doi.org/10.1111/jabr.12124.
Yagin FH, de Fernandes MSS. The importance of medical terminology in the health sector. JESPAR. 2024;2(1):132–6. https://doi.org/10.5281/zenodo.11544933.

Yarnitsky D. Conditioned pain modulation (the diffuse noxious inhibitory control-like effect): its relevance for acute and chronic pain states. Curr Opin Anesthesiol. 2010;23:611–5. https://doi.org/10.1097/ACO.0b013e32833c348b.

Yarnitsky D, Arendt-Nielsen L, Bouhassira D, Edwards RR, Fillingim RB, Granot M, Hansson P, Lautenbacher S, Marchand S, Wilder-Smith O. Recommendations on terminology and practice of psychophysical DNIC testing. Eur J Pain. 2010;14:339. https://doi.org/10.1016/j.ejpain.2010.02.004.

Case Studies in Tautology, Circular Reasoning and Conflation: Fibromyalgia and Myofascial Pain "Syndromes"

Abstract The problems in language and reasoning discussed in chapter "Errors in Language and Logic Call for Epistemic Discipline" are exemplified in the literature concerning the widely prevalent clinical problem of chronic musculoskeletal pain for which there is no obvious source of nociception. This chapter examines two popular constructs that seek to account for the clinical phenomena: "fibrositis" and its sequel "fibromyalgia syndrome", and "myofascial pain syndrome".

This is not another treatise on the clinical problems themselves but a dissection of the epistemological traps into which these constructs have fallen. It is shown how both are mired in conflation and circular reasoning, resulting in them being so broad as to accommodate all possibilities, thus constituting tautologies. In effect, this makes it impossible not to apply either or both "labels" in any clinical situation of musculoskeletal pain of uncertain nature.

Theorists of both "fibromyalgia" and "myofascial pain" constructs have succumbed to conflating pain and nociception, have failed to distinguish cause from effect and have needed to invoke comorbidity with other pain conditions in order to provide coherence for their constructs. Meanwhile, the observed clinical phenomena demand explanation in neuroscientific terms, the "elephant-in-the-room" being the key clinical phenomenon of allodynia, which reflects the salient role of nociception in pain experiences. As will be shown, this moves the focus of the argument from presumed concrete entities to dynamic neurophysiological processes.

Conflation, Circular Reasoning and Tautology

A particular arena is which epistemic discipline is required is that of pain experienced in musculoskeletal tissues for which there is no obvious lesion or, more specifically, an identifiable origin of nociception. The case-load and cost to the individual and to society world-wide of this problem is enormous (Gill et al. 2023).

This Handbook is not the place to discuss the epidemiology, biology or sociology of chronic musculoskeletal pain. However, two constructs that have sought to explain, if not also to exploit, the phenomena provide case studies into faulty

M. Cohen, J. Quintner, *A Philosophical Handbook for Pain Medicine Practice*,
https://doi.org/10.1007/978-981-92-1682-6_9

reasoning, which is one of this book's main philosophical themes. Those constructs are "fibromyalgia syndrome" and "myofascial pain syndrome".

It must be emphasised at the outset that the clinical phenomena that these constructs have sought to explain are not in dispute. What is of concern here is how this clinical problem of chronic musculoskeletal pain has been refracted through modern biomedical thinking, without achieving satisfaction for either experiencers or observers.

This chapter is not another attempt to explain the phenomena—although a pathway to resolution of frustration is offered—but a dissection of the epistemological traps into which these constructs have fallen. Each construct has a huge literature in which the same errors continue to be perpetuated. That in itself is an illustration of the illusory truth effect mentioned in chapter "Errors in Language and Logic Call for Epistemic Discipline".

Many examples of conflation and circular reasoning have been given in this Handbook.

To recapitulate some definitions:

Conflation

Conflation is a fallacy which occurs when distinct things are treated as if they were the same, leading to confusion and potentially flawed reasoning. The outcome of conflation has been called "an undifferentiated smudge" (Haught 1995).

In the current context, an example is the conflation of the "trigger points" of myofascial pain syndrome and the "tender points" of fibromyalgia syndrome:

> The widespread spontaneous pain pattern in fibromyalgia (FM) is a summation of multiple regional pains due to active MTrPs [myofascial trigger points]. A regional pain in FM is from local active MTrPs and/or referred from remote active MTrPs. Positive tender points specified in FM are MTrPs, either active or latent (Ge 2010).

Circular Reasoning

Circular reasoning is a logical fallacy where an argument's conclusion is used as its own proof. For examples, fibromyalgia has been promoted as "a common and recognisable cause of chronic diffuse musculoskeletal pain" (Goldenberg (1995), and "myofascial pain is a common cause of acute and chronic pain" (Lam et al. 2024). These examples also illustrate confusion of cause and effect.

Tautology

A tautology in logic is a proposition that is true under all possible circumstances or interpretations. For example, "tender points are inherently more tender than non-tender points, whether one is dealing with normal or fibromyalgia patients" (Tunks et al. 1988).

Antecedents to Fibromyalgia Syndrome and Myofascial Pain Syndrome

The phenomena of muscle pain and tenderness in the absence of obvious disease have been well recognised for a long time but remain incompletely understood. These problems attracted labels such as muscular rheumatism, neurasthenia and fibrositis, themselves models of disease based on speculation regarding somatic pathology. When underlying pathology could not be found, they tended to fall foul of dualistic thinking and psychogenic pathogenesis was preferred (Quintner and Cohen 1994a, b; Cohen and Quintner 1996; Quintner and Cohen 1999). This is discussed further below.

The most developed of these models was "fibrositis", a term proposed by the neurologist Sir William Gowers (1904). The main feature of "fibrositis" was the presence in soft tissues (fat, musculotendinous structures and nerve sheaths) of localised "trigger points" that were tender and from which pain could radiate or apparently be induced elsewhere. The phenomenon was thought to be secondary to recent or previous infections. When palpable, these points were referred to as "fibrositic nodules" (Stockman 1920; Copeman 1936, 1943).

During the late 1930s, it was postulated that palpable muscle hardenings could set up a reflexly induced increase in muscle tension resulting in a "pain-reflex-pain self-perpetuating cycle" that could be disrupted by ethyl chloride sprayed onto the overlying skin or by local injections (Kraus, cited by Simons 1975). This was the "vicious circle" hypothesis favoured by pioneers in pain theory.

Fibromyalgia Syndrome

Early Evolution

In 1992, the "Copenhagen declaration" proclaimed the establishment of fibromyalgia syndrome (FMS) as a distinctive diagnosis, defined as a "painful, non-articular condition predominantly involving muscles" and as the "commonest cause of chronic widespread, musculoskeleletal pain" (Anon. 1992). Thus, a pain syndrome was said to cause itself—the ultimate in circular argument (Cohen and Quintner 1993).

"Fibromyalgia" was first conceived as a diagnosis in the 1970s (Smythe and Moldofsky 1977; Smythe 1979; Yunus et al. 1981), to describe a syndrome characterised by widespread pain and increased sensitivity to pressure at various specific anatomical locations known as "tender points". These tender sites were considered to be integral to the diagnosis but were mostly unknown to the patient and, inexplicably, unrelated to the pain (Quintner and Cohen 1999). Over this period, there was a series of proposed diagnostic criteria, all relying on tender points (in the absence of any clinicopathological explanation), as well as adding in non-musculoskeletal features such as sleep disturbance, fatigue, headache, altered mood and irritable bowel symptoms, culminating in the classification criteria published in 1990 by the American College of Rheumatology (ACR criteria), which were purported to distinguish FMS from other rheumatic conditions (Wolfe et al. 1990).

These ACR 1990 criteria for FMS were widespread chronic[1] pain and "tenderness" at any 11 of 18 defined musculoskeletal sites ("tender points"). Three issues arose from that study (Cohen and Quintner 1993, 1998; Quintner and Cohen 1999):

(i) 19% of the defining population had the required number of tender points but were considered not to have FMS (the false-positive rate). There has been no answer to the question, what condition did these patients have?
(ii) What condition did patients with widespread pain but fewer than 11 tender points have? Provided that other so-called characteristic (non-musculoskeletal) symptoms were present, the diagnosis could still be awarded to these patients.
(iii) What was the diagnosis for people with a high tender point count but without widespread pain?

Tender points were found in the general population to be associated with psychological and general distress, independently of pain status (Croft et al. 1994). It was also found that that there was no correlation between any symptom or combination of symptoms with the presence, number or sensitivity of tender points (Quimby et al. 1988). Furthermore, it was later stated that there is no discrete boundary between FMS and non-FMS, thus negating the tender point count criterion (Wolfe 1997). Taken together with another assertion that fibromyalgia may co-exist with "any other condition" (Wolfe et al. 1990), how would it ever be possible not to "diagnose" FMS in any person presenting with sole remaining criterion of "widespread pain"?

Thus, this construct of FMS constituted a tautology, as it included all possibilities (Cohen and Quintner 1993), and as such lacked explanatory power and therefore diagnostic and therapeutic utility. In effect, FMS became a synonym for widespread pain.

[1] Pain of at least 3 months duration, consistent with the IASP definition.

Later Evolution

The necessary discarding of the tender point count criterion had two major consequences. Firstly, the cardinal clinical clue to the biology of FMS—tenderness or, more correctly, mechanical allodynia—was ignored in the diagnostic process. Secondly, recourse was taken to quantifying the non-pain-related features said to be "characteristic" of FMS, even though the "syndrome" itself remained undefined.[2]

In 2010, a new diagnostic approach to FMS was suggested, consisting of:

(a) a "widespread pain index (WPI)", or in how many specified body regions was pain being experienced, with a range from 0 to 19; and
(b) a "symptom severity scale (SSS)", based on how many and how severe were the three symptom domains of fatigue, sleep disturbance and cognitive difficulties, with a score range from 0 to 12.

A diagnosis of FMS could be made if:

(i) WPI+SSS $\geq$ 13, or
WPI$\geq$7 + SSS$\geq$5, or
WPI 3-6 + SSS$\geq$9; and
(ii) There was no "disorder that would otherwise explain the pain" (Wolfe et al. 2010; Russell 2011).

It should be noted that this "diagnosis by numbers" relied solely on patient report.

In 2016, this approach was modified, to require, for a diagnosis of FMS:

(a) generalised pain, defined as pain in at least 4 of 5 regions; and
(b) symptoms to have been present at a similar level for at least 3 months; and
(c) WPI $\geq$ 7 + SSS $\geq$ 5 or WPI 4–6 + SSS $\geq$ 9;

qualified by

> "A diagnosis of fibromyalgia is valid irrespective of other diagnoses. A diagnosis of fibromyalgia does not exclude the presence of other clinically important illnesses" (Wolfe et al. 2016).

This remained "diagnosis by numbers", the main change being from "widespread" pain to "generalised" pain. It was claimed that this revision allowed the criteria to function for both diagnostic and classification purposes, with the caveats that the physician-based criteria were valid for individual patient diagnosis, while the self-report version was not valid for individual clinical diagnosis but was valid for research studies (Wolfe et al. 2016).

The most recent iteration of this approach (Arnold et al. 2019) noted that, after almost three decades of investigation, there was no gold-standard definition of FMS

---

[2] Strictly speaking, FMS and indeed MPS were never "syndromes" but rather "symptom clusters". Syndrome implies that the various components share common mechanisms; symptom cluster reflects only concurrence of components. As an analogy, constellations appearing in the night sky may appear to be close (~syndromes) but are in fact light years apart (~clusters).

and, therefore, there was no agreement on prevalence of the condition. These authors took the view that FMS should be identified as "predominantly a chronic pain disorder" (*sic*) and proposed a first core criterion of "multisite" pain—to be distinguished from "widespread" and "generalised" pain as described above—defined as pain in 6 or more sites of a possible 9 (as indicated on a body chart). The second core criterion was a step backwards from the preceding "associated symptoms" approach, identifying only "moderate to severe sleep problems or fatigue". In a classical example of circular argument, fatigue was "defined as physical or mental fatigue judged as at least moderate severity by the health care professional".

It was claimed that "... the presence of [multisite pain] in combination with moderate to severe fatigue or sleep problems was sufficient to identify the FM patients. This simplified the criteria so that no scoring of associated symptoms was required" (Arnold et al. 2019, p. 621). However, "tenderness", "dyscognition", musculoskeletal "stiffness" and "environmental sensitivity or hypervigilance" were considered to "support" a diagnosis of FMS. Furthermore, the authors maintained these qualifying statements from previous iterations: "... comorbid disorders, including other chronic pain disorders, are common in patients with FM"; and "the presence of other disorders does not necessarily exclude a diagnosis of FM".

All these formulations of FMS, which persist to the present, perpetuate the epistemological errors of circular argument and of confusion between symptom cluster and syndrome. They also illustrate the fallacy that the evidence that leads to a conclusion cannot be then used to justify the veracity of that conclusion (Medawar 1969).

In this context, it is again worth noting that FMS has been put forward as the "prototype" of "primary" musculoskeletal pain (Fitzcharles et al. 2022) and of nociplastic pain in the musculoskeletal system (Kosek et al. 2021), reflecting the conflation of clinical, taxonomic and mechanistic concepts, as discussed in chapter "The Salient Role of Nociception".

FMS remains a clinical pseudodiagnosis for the complaint of chronic widespread or generalised or multisite pain and as such remains a tautology. This situation will persist until the diagnostic link to clinical evidence of altered nociceptive function that underpins the phenomenon of tenderness (allodynia[3]) is restored and properly established (Cohen and Quintner 1993; Cohen et al. 2023; Weisman et al. 2025).

Myofascial Pain Syndrome

Myofascial Pain Theory

An earlier but ultimately parallel evolution from "fibrositis" is the construct of "myofascial pain" (Travell and Rinzler 1952). This claim recalled the "vicious cycle" theory mentioned above, attributed to "trigger areas in myofascial

[3] See chapter "Translation into the Clinic".

structures". This culminated in the 1963 articulation of "myofascial pain syndrome", the theory of which comprised two essential components: (i) the trigger point, a localised area of tenderness or hyperirritability deep within voluntary muscle; and (ii) a predictable discrete zone of deep aching pain, which could be located in the immediate region of, or remote from, the trigger point, and which was worsened by palpation of it (Travell and Simons 1983).

Such "trigger points" (previously known as "fibrositic nodules") were said:

- to develop within every voluntary muscle and in multiple locations within a given muscle;
- to vary in location from person to person; and
- to be located in "palpable taut bands", which represented shortened muscle fibres which in turn were said to be a potential source of peripheral nerve entrapment.

To explain pain in muscles that lacked obvious trigger points, myofascial pain theory postulated the "latent" trigger point, which was said to be a site of tenderness within a muscle, unassociated with spontaneous pain but having the potential to be activated by any of a myriad of factors within or without the body.

To explain the tendency for localised muscle pain to become widespread, myofascial pain theory claimed that "active" trigger points could in some unspecified way self-propagate to become "secondary" trigger points in other muscles and even to "metastasise" throughout the bodily musculature.

Lastly, myofascial pain theory asserted that trigger points could be found in other (non-myofascial) tissues including skin, scar tissue, fascia, ligaments and periosteum.

In essence, myofascial pain theory claims that "myofascial pain" is caused by painful loci in myofascial tissues, which constitutes a classical circular argument. Furthermore, through the metaphysics of "trigger points"—active, latent, secondary and metastatic—all non-visceral pain can be explained. This again constitutes a tautology, a proposition so broad that it includes all possibilities, and thus lacks explanatory power, certainly in scientific and clinical senses.

Myofascial Pain as a Case Study for Refutation of Theory

The theory of regional (or widespread) pain based on myofascial trigger points was fundamentally a biomedical conjecture. It postulated a somatic lesion that was the origin of nociception, although it was never stated in such terms, as it confused pain as cause and as effect. It did provide an opportunity however to apply falsifiability as a test for the validity of a theory. This exercise turned on whether actual—not latent or secondary—trigger points could be identified, in order to determine what relationship they might have to nociception, and therefore possibly to a pain experience.

The trigger point conjecture has been comprehensively refuted on the following grounds (Quintner et al. 2015; Quintner and Cohen 2016):

1. Clinical examination

An extensive review identified at least 19 different sets of diagnostic criteria used for the MPS/trigger point syndrome, and found a lack of consistency and consensus on case definition (Tough et al. 2007). A similar study concluded, "On the basis of the limited number of studies available, and significant problems with their design, reporting, statistical integrity, and clinical applicability, physical examination cannot currently be recommended as a reliable test for the diagnosis of TPs" (Lucas et al. 2009:80).

In other words, physical examination cannot be relied upon to diagnose a condition that is said to be defined by that physical examination. By that criterion alone, the conjecture should have been rejected.

2. Search for a lesion

No plausible let alone consistent anatomical, histological, biochemical or electromyographical pathology has been found in tissue taken from putative trigger points.

3. Evidence from "treatment" of trigger points

Non-invasive therapy interventions advocated for myofascial pain syndrome include "spray and stretch", transcutaneous electrical stimulation (TENS), massage and high-power ultrasound (Chen et al. 2001). Invasive treatments have included local injections of anaesthetic agents, injection of corticosteroids, injections of botulinum toxin, needle acupuncture and dry needling (Lavelle et al. 2007). Systematic reviews have been unable to find evidence of any effectiveness of most interventions beyond placebo effect (Cummings and White 2001; Rickards 2006; Tough et al. 2007; Annaswamy et al. 2011).

Despite its refutation, myofascial pain theory continues to be promoted (Phan et al. 2020; Cao et al. 2021; Fernández-de-las-Peñas et al. 2023).

Both "Tender Points" and "Trigger Points" Miss the Point

Refutation of a theory in the case of myofascial pain and rejection of a crude "point count" in the case of fibromyalgia do not detract from acknowledging the existence of the clinical phenomena that these constructs sought to explain.

For a long time, the "trigger points" of myofascial pain syndrome and the "tender points" of fibromyalgia syndrome have been confused or conflated (Wolfe et al. 1992; Ge 2010). A typical example, one that also conflates theories of pathophysiology, is:

> On the one hand, in fact, TrPs [trigger points] are more frequent in FMS [fibromyalgia] due to a higher susceptibility in FMS to microtraumatic events that are recognized (*sic*) causative factors for TrP formation. On the other hand, muscle TrPs in any individual represent a powerful peripheral source of nociceptive impulses; in time, these are likely to favor the development of central sensitization phenomena that can promote the clinical manifestation of FMS [that is, tender points] in predisposed individuals. (Giamberardino et al. 2011)

More recently, an attempt was made to resurrect myofascial pain syndrome in the context of reconceptualising "chronic primary musculoskeletal pain" as "regional fibromyalgia" (Fitzcharles et al. 2022), another example of conflating a taxonomic category with a clinical symptom cluster. It has also been asserted that:

> ... myofascial TrP pain is fundamentally a nociceptive pain condition, and should not be classified primarily as neuropathic pain, but can be classified as nociplastic pain when it has features consistent with central sensitization, and can be part of a predominantly neuropathic or nociplastic pain condition as a comorbid disorder. (Fernández-de-las-Peñas et al. 2023:5)

The tautology here is inescapable, reminiscent of the claim that fibromyalgia can be co-morbid with any other chronic pain condition.

The "points" in question have no structural basis and therefore cannot be sites of activation of nociceptors. Their "tenderness"—strictly, mechanical allodynia—can only reflect a sensitised nociceptive apparatus.[4] This proposal, in each of these two contexts, invoking the physiological phenomenon of "secondary hyperalgesia", is not new (Cohen and Quintner 1993; Quintner and Cohen 1994a).

Epistemological Overview: Why This Apparent Impasse?

Although the constructs of FMS and MPS have been shown to be tautologies and thus to lack explanatory power, both are rooted in the biomedical model and emerged in the mid-twentieth century at a time when psychogenic theories for unexplained medical conditions were popular. Smythe, an early advocate of FMS, explicitly tried to quarantine patients with diffuse musculoskeletal pain and tenderness away from implications of psychogenesis (Smythe 1979). Indeed, the fundamental consideration that nociception is necessary for pain demands that a somatic cause be found for the clinical phenomena under consideration here.

Thus, we have an impasse in which neither school of thought has been able to escape circular reasoning. The myofascial pain theorists continue to adhere to a doctrine that insists that there is local peripheral nociception, despite overwhelming evidence to the contrary. The fibromyalgia theorists appear to accept that increased central nociceptive function underlies the phenomena but have retreated from dissecting "tenderness" towards invoking features that are unrelated to nociception, succeeding only in conflating their chameleonic symptom cluster with "nociplastic pain".

Both sets of theorists succumbed to conflating pain and nociception, failing to distinguish cause from effect, and having to invoke comorbidity with "other" pain conditions in order to provide coherence for their constructs. Contributing to this confusion lies the linguistic problem that the so-called "pain descriptors"—nociceptive, neuropathic and nociplastic—are in fact hypotheses of nociception. This is

[4] See chapters "The Salient Role of Nociception" and "Translation into the Clinic".

despite the unequivocal statement that pain and nociception are different phenomena. As has been argued in this volume, this in turn reflects paradoxes discoverable in the definition of pain (Chapter "Clarifying the Definition of Pain") and persistence of the aphorism that nociception is not necessary for pain (Chapter "The Salient Role of Nociception").

At another level of analysis, these constructs invoked the substantialist ontology that dominates Western philosophy. That is to say, there are always things (substances) to be found to explain phenomena. This view focusses on static existence. That has tended to obscure other explanatory pathways, namely that phenomena reflect dynamic change (processes or properties) rather than static existence. In these cases, the focus was on "points", be they "tender" or "trigger", rather than on processes that might underlie nociception and pain.

A Historical Note

The vagueness inherent in the constructs of FMS and MPS, especially the former, continues to hold open a door to those who would still favour a psychogenic pathogenesis. This was exemplified by the historian Edward Shorter who wrote that FMS was "... heaven-sent to doctors as a diagnostic label for pain patients who display an important neurotic component in their illness" (Shorter 1992), reflecting the body-mind dualistic thinking that had shaped the medical interpretation of these phenomena over the last two centuries.

In the eighteenth century, ideas of "hysteria", "hypochondria" and "melancholy" became conflated with known diseases of the brain and nerves. The new terms *nervousness*, *neurasthenia* and, later, *neurosis* evolved during the nineteenth century to denote the concept that affections of the mind were indeed disorders of the brain.

However, over a critical 30-year period from 1890 to 1920, "neurosis" was redefined by physicians from being an organic disorder of the nervous system to "psychoneurosis", implying an entirely psychogenic pathogenesis (Quintner and Cohen 1994b). This reflected resurfacing of body-mind confusion, an epistemological error which has had a profound effect on subsequent clinical formulations of many pain syndromes.

For example, in the nineteenth century, the pathophysiology of diffuse spinal pain following trauma was the subject of a heated debate between proponents of somatic and psychological theories. This debate was played out against a background of personal injury compensation for those injured in railway accidents. The term "railway spine" reflected the views of those who favoured a somatic insult, but this rapidly evolved into the term "railway brain", favouring the view that the insult was psychic (Cohen and Quintner 1996). This evolution also resulted in conditions previously regarded as somatic, such as the craft palsies (including the various forms of "writer's cramp"), acquiring a psychogenic connotation. This persisted into the 1980s, in the case of painful neck and upper limb disorders acquired in an occupational context, known in Australia as "repetition strain injuries" or "RSI" (Quintner and Cohen 1994b).[5]

These conceptual difficulties and the ensuing vigorous arguments over nosology have obscured the quest to explain the observed clinical phenomena in neuroscientific terms, the "elephant-in-the-room" being the key clinical phenomenon of allodynia (Chapter "Translation into the Clinic"), reflecting the salient role of nociception in pain (Chapter "The Salient Role of Nociception").

References

Annaswamy TM, De Luigi AJ, O'Neill BJ, Keole N, Berbrayer D. Emerging concepts in the treatment of myofascial pain: a review of medications, modalities, and needle-based interventions. PM R. 2011;3:940–61. https://doi.org/10.1016/j.pmrj.2011.06.013.

Anon. Fibromyalgia: the Copenhagen declaration. Lancet. 1992;340:663–4.

Arnold LM, Bennett RM, Crofford LJ, Dean LE, Clauw DJ, Goldenberg DL, Fitzcharles M-A, Paiva ES, Staud R, Sarzi-Puttini P, Buskila D, Macfarlane GJ. AAPT diagnostic criteria for fibromyalgia. J Pain. 2019;20(6):611–28. https://doi.org/10.1016/j.jpain.2018.10.008.

Cao QW, Peng BG, Wang L, Huang YQ, Jia DL, Jiang H, Lv Y, Liu XG, Liu RG, Li Y, Song T, Shen W, Yu LZ, Zheng YJ, Liu YQ, Huang D. Expert consensus on the diagnosis and treatment of myofascial pain syndrome. World J Clin Cases. 2021;9:2077–89.

Chen JT, Chung KC, Hou CR, et al. Inhibitory effect of dry needling on the spontaneous electrical activity recorded from myofascial trigger spots of rabbit skeletal muscle. Am J Phys Med Rehabil. 2001;80:729–35. https://doi.org/10.1097/00002060-200110000-00004.

Cohen ML, Quintner JL. Fibromyalgia syndrome, a problem of tautology. Lancet. 1993;342:906–9. https://doi.org/10.1016/0140-6736(93)91950-q.

Cohen ML, Quintner JL. The derailment of railway spine: a timely lesson for post-traumatic fibromyalgia. Pain Rev. 1996;3:181–222.

Cohen ML, Quintner JL. Fibromyalgia syndrome and disability: a failed construct fails those in pain. Med J Aust. 1998;168:402–4.

Cohen ML, Quintner JL, Weisman A. "Nociplastic pain": a challenge to nosology and to nociception. J Pain. 2023;24(12):2131–39. https://doi.org/10.1016/j.pain.2023.07.019.

Copeman WS. Treatment of fibrositis. Brit Med J. 1936;1:1219–20.

Copeman WS. A clinical contribution to the study of the fibrositic nodule. Ann Rheum Dis. 1943;3:222–6.

Croft P, Schollum J, Silman P. Population study of tender point counts and pain as evidence of fibromyalgia. Brit Med J. 1994;309:96–9. https://doi.org/10.1136/bmj.309.6956.696.

Cummings TM, White AR. Needling therapies in the management of myofascial trigger point pain: a systematic review. Arch Phys Med Rehabil. 2001;82:986–92. https://doi.org/10.1053/apmr.2001.24023.

Fernández-de-las-Peñas C, Nijs J, Cagnie B, Gerwin RD, Plaza-Manzano G, Valera-Calero JA, Arendt-Nielsen L. Myofascial pain syndrome: a nociceptive condition comorbid with neuropathic or nociplastic pain. Life. 2023;13:694. https://doi.org/10.3390/life13030694.

[5] Another example of this evolution from "neurosis" to "psychoneurosis" in a non-pain context was that of shell-shock in World War I, connoted initially as *"commotio cerebri"* but then as *"emotio cerebri"*. See Quintner and Cohen 1994b.

Fitzcharles M-A, Cohen SP, Clauw DJ, Littlejohn G, Usui C, Häuser W. Chronic primary musculoskeletal pain: a new concept of non-structural regional pain. Pain Rep. 2022;7:e1024. https://doi.org/10.1097/PR9.0000000000001024.
Ge HY. Prevalence of myofascial trigger points in fibromyalgia: the overlap of two common problems. Curr Pain Headache Rep. 2010;14:339–45. https://doi.org/10.1007/s11916-010-0127-5.
Giamberardino MA, Affaitati G, Fabrizio A, Constantini R. Effect of treatment of myofascial trigger points on the pain of fibromyalgia. Curr Pain Headache Rep. 2011;15:393–9. https://doi.org/10.1007/s11916-011-0205-3.
Gill TK, Mittinty MM, March LM, Steinmetz JD, Culbreth GT, Cross M, Kopec JA, Woolf AD, Haile LM, Hagins H, Ong KL. Global, regional, and national burden of other musculoskeletal disorders, 1990–2020, and projections to 2050: a systematic analysis of the Global Burden of Disease Study 2021. Lancet Rheumatol. 2023;5(11):e670–82.
Goldenberg DL. Fibromyalgia: why such controversy? Ann Rheum Dis. 1995;54:3–5. https://doi.org/10.1136/ard.54.1.3.
Gowers WR. Lumbago: its lessons and analogues. Brit Med J. 1904;1:117–21.
Haught JF. Science and religion: from conflict to conversation. New York: Paulist Press; 1995.
Kosek E, Clauw D, Nijs J, Baron R, Gilron I, Harris RE, Mico J-A, Rice ACS, Sterling M. Chronic nociplastic pain affecting the musculoskeletal system: clinical criteria and grading system. Pain. 2021;162:2629–34. https://doi.org/10.1097/j.pain.0000000000002324.
Lam C, Francio VT, Gustafson K, Carroll M, York A, Chadwick AL. Myofascial pain – a major player in musculoskeletal pain. Best Pract Res Clin Rheumatol. 2024;38:101944. https://doi.org/10.1016/j.berh.2024.101944.
Lavelle ED, Lavelle W, Smith HS. Myofascial trigger points. Anesthesiol Clin. 2007;25:841–51. https://doi.org/10.1016/j.anclin.2007.07.003.
Lucas N, Macaskill P, Irwig L, Moran R, Bogduk N. Reliability of physical examination for diagnosis of myofascial trigger points: a systematic review of the literature. Clin J Pain. 2009;25:80–9. https://doi.org/10.1097/AJP.0b013e31817e13b6.
Medawar P. Induction and intuition in scientific thought. London: Methuen; 1969.
Phan V, Shah J, Tandon H, Srbely J, DeStefano S, Khumbare D, Sikdar S, Clouse A, Gandhi A, Gerber L. Myofascial pain syndrome: a narrative review identifying inconsistencies in nomenclature. PM R. 2020;12:916–25. https://doi.org/10.1002/pmrj.12290.
Quimby LG, Block SR, Gratwick GM. Fibromyalgia: generalized pain intolerence and manifold symptoms reporting. J Rheumatol. 1988;15(8):1264–70.
Quintner JL, Cohen ML. Referred pain of peripheral nerve origin: an alternative to the "myofascial pain" construct. Clin J Pain. 1994a;10:243–51.
Quintner JL, Cohen ML. Occupation neuroses and the psychogenic connotation of "repetition strain injury": the misconstruction of neurosis. Integ Psychiatr. 1994b;10:165–76.
Quintner J, Cohen ML. Fibromyalgia falls foul of a fallacy. Lancet. 1999;353:1092–4. https://doi.org/10.1016/S0140-6736(98)06468-X.
Quintner JL, Cohen ML. The challenge of validating the experience of chronic pain: the importance of intersubjectivity and reframing. In: Van Rysewyck S, editors. Meanings of Pain. Springer International Publishing AG; 2016. pp. 281–93.
Quintner J, Bove G, Cohen M. A critical evaluation of the "trigger point" phenomenon. Rheumatology. 2015;54:392–9. https://doi.org/10.1093/rheumatology/keu471.
Rickards LD. The effectiveness of non-invasive treatments for active myofascial trigger point pain: a systematic review of the literature. Int J Osteopathic Med. 2006;9:120–36.
Russell IJ. Future perspectives in generalised musculoskeletal pain syndromes. Best Pract Res Clin Rheumatol. 2011;25:321–31. https://doi.org/10.1016/j.berh.2011.03.003.
Shorter E. From paralysis to fatigue. New York: The Free Press; 1992. p. 295–323.
Simons DG. Muscle pain syndromes, Part I. American J. Phys Med. 1975;54:289–311.
Smythe HA. "Fibrositis" as a disorder of pain modulation. Clin Rheum Dis. 1979;5:823–32.
Smythe HA, Moldofsky H. Two contributions to understanding of the "fibrositis" syndrome. Bull Rheum Dis. 1977;28(1):928–31.

Stockman R. Rheumatism and Arthritis. Edinburgh: W Green & Son; 1920.

Tough EA, White AR, Richards S, Campbell J. Variability of criteria used to diagnose myofascial trigger point pain syndrome—evidence from a review of the literature. Clin J Pain. 2007;23:278–86. https://doi.org/10.1097/AJP.0b013e31802fda7c.

Travell J, Rinzler SH. The myofascial genesis of pain. Post-Grad Med. 1952;11(5):425–34.

Travell JG, Simons DG. Myofascial pain and dysfunction: the trigger point manual. Baltimore: Williams and Wilkins; 1983.

Tunks E, Crook J, Norman G, Kalaher S. Tender points in fibromyalgia. Pain. 1988;34:11–9. https://doi.org/10.1016/0304-3959(88)90176-5.

Weisman A, Quintner J, Cohen M. Adieu to an aphorism: nocicpetion is necessary but not sufficient for pain. Brain. 2025;149(2):422–31. https://doi.org/10.1093/brain/awaf387. Published online October 2025

Wolfe F. The relation between tender points and fibromyalgia symptom variables: evidence that fibromyalgia is not a discrete disorder in the clinic. Ann Rheum Dis. 1997;56:268–71. https://doi.org/10.1136/ard.56.4.268.

Wolfe F, Smythe HA, Yunus MB, Bennett RM, Bombadier C, Goldenberg DL, et al. The American College of Rheumatology criteria for the classification of fibromyalgia. Arthritis Rheum. 1990;33(2):160–72. https://doi.org/10.1002/art.1780330203.

Wolfe F, Simons DG, Fricton J, Bennett RM, Goldenberg DL, Gerwin R, Hathaway D, McCain GA, Russell IJ, Sanders HO, et al. The fibromyalgia and myofascial pain syndromes: a preliminary study of tender points and trigger points in persons with fibromyalgia, myofascial pain syndrome and no disease. J Rheumatol. 1992;19(6):944–51.

Wolfe F, Clauw DJ, Fitzcharles M-A, Goldenberg DL, Katz PS, Mease P, et al. The American College of Rheumatology preliminary diagnostic criteria for fibromyalgia and measurement of symptom severity. Arth Care Res. 2010;62(5):600–10. https://doi.org/10.1002/acr.20140.

Wolfe F, Clauw DJ, Fitzcharles M-A, Goldenberg DL, Häuser W, Katz RL. Revision to the 2010/2011 fibromyalgia diagnsotic criteria. Semin Arthritis Rheum. 2016;46(3):319–29. https://doi.org/10.1016/j.semarthrit.2016.08.012.

Yunus M, Masi AT, Calabro JJ, Miler KA, Feigenbaum SL. Primary fibromyalgia (fibrositis): clinical study of 50 patients with matched normal controls. Semin Arthritis Rheum. 1981;11:151–71. https://doi.org/10.1016/0049-0172(81)90096-2.

Translation into the Clinic

Abstract In this Chapter, further clinical implications of the three main philosophical themes identified in this Handbook are explored.

Under the theme of the salient role of nociception in the pain experience, the key phenomenon of clinical allodynia is discussed, defined here as pain in response to a non-noxious stimulus. The history of the psychophysical terms allodynia and hyperalgesia is presented, and the divergence in their usage between the experimental and clinical perspectives is held responsible for the confusion that exists in the literature. Allodynia, whether spontaneously reported or specifically induced, is asserted as being the fundamental clinical clue to the state of activation of the nociceptive apparatus.

The theme of the inherent uncertainty, for experiencer and observer alike, of the meaning of the pain experience has focussed on the two-person encounter in the clinical intersubjective space. Here, two (of many possible) perturbations of that encounter that can compromise validation of both parties are explored. These are stigmatisation as a withdrawal of empathy and misinformation as violation of trust.

The chapter then returns to the theme of epistemic discipline that has pervaded this Handbook. Unclear, inaccurate or illogical usage of terms and constructs has been held responsible for many of the barriers encountered in the field of Pain Medicine. The particular discussion here is towards a new nomenclature for clinical pain problems, especially in the somatic dimension, in a multiaxial formulation matrix.

As has been emphasised, this Handbook is intended first and foremost to be an invitation to "how one might think about the issue" rather than a definitive "how to deal with the issue" in the practice of Pain Medicine.

Three main themes have emerged:

- the need for epistemic discipline, which means taking care to ensure that words and concepts are being used correctly, in accordance with clarity of definition, accuracy of information and principles of logic;

M. Cohen, J. Quintner, *A Philosophical Handbook for Pain Medicine Practice*,
https://doi.org/10.1007/978-981-92-1682-6_10

- the centrality of nociception to the pain experience ("nociception is necessary but not sufficient for pain"); and
- the inherent uncertainty, for experiencer and observer alike, of the meaning of the pain experience.

Of these themes, the first is pervasive in the pain-related literature, of which many examples have been given and their clinical implications presented. In this Chapter, further translation into the clinic of the second and third themes is explored, before returning to the first theme in a discussion of diagnostic formulation.

The Pivotal Role of Nociception

Implications of Reconceptualising Nociception

In chapter "The Salient Role of Nociception", it was argued that nociception is necessary but not sufficient for pain, contingent on a reformulation of nociception that broadens that construct from "the neural process of encoding noxious stimuli" to "activation of a nociceptive apparatus". Here, "nociceptive" means "capable of encoding noxious stimuli", thus maintaining the logical and lexical consistency of the IASP terminology.[1]

The very term "nociception" implies a process that has been activated. It follows that "activated nociception" is a truism. By contrast, to talk about "activation of nociceptors" or "activation of a nociceptive apparatus" is accurate usage.

This reconceptualisation of nociception has two major implications. The first is that all pain, especially chronic pain, is potentially explicable at a biological (somatic) level. This makes untenable the view that non-somatic factors—psychological or social—*cause* pain, because they do not involve nociception. In other words, psychological and/or social factors are neither necessary nor sufficient for a pain experience. This does not deny the influence of such factors on modifying that experience or the importance of considering these dimensions on a par with the "biological" or somatic dimension in a clinical biopsychosocial conceptual framework.[2]

The second is that the metaphorical use of "pain" to denote suffering can be parsed according to whether or not that complaint is attributable to nociception. This distinction has only recently come under closer scrutiny, as discussed in chapter "Trying to Gain Traction on a Slippery Subject". Not all pain experiences are necessarily associated with suffering and not all suffering in a person experiencing pain may be due to nociception. In turn, this also has major clinical implications, as it is incumbent upon the health professional not only to recognise suffering but also to determine to what that might be attributable. Not all complaints of "pain" may

[1] Available at https://www.iasp-pain.org/resources/terminology/

[2] See also Chapter "Conceptual Frameworks".

have a somatic origin but an expanded concept of nociception would confer validation for many of those people whose pain is often labelled as "medically unexplained". This is in fact embraced in the recent construct of "nociplastic" pain, which is not a label of exclusion but requires clinical evidence to suggest that nociception has been engaged in the absence of "nociceptive" or "neuropathic" processes.[3]

Thus, the principle captured by the revised aphorism, "nociception is necessary but not sufficient for pain", can be seen to fundamentally reset clinical assessment of the somatic (or "biological") dimension of the biopsychosocial framework and the therapeutic approaches to that, without detracting at all from the importance of the psychological and social dimensions. This would also serve to realign research activity with clinical aspects, to focus on nociception on the one hand and on distinguishing pain from suffering on the other, with clear therapeutic implications at both individual and public health levels.

Clinical Allodynia as a Key Phenomenon

The Cardinal Clinical Issue of "Tenderness"

The starting point is the clinical human report of two phenomena:

(i) (increased) pain in response to a stimulus that "normally" induces pain; and
(ii) pain induced by a stimulus that "normally" does not do so.

Both these phenomena are captured in the lay term "tenderness".[4]

Technically, phenomenon (i) is termed "hyperalgesia", while phenomenon (ii) is termed "allodynia". The current IASP definitions of these terms are:

- ALLODYNIA is pain due to a stimulus that does not normally provoke pain.
- HYPERALGESIA is increased pain from a stimulus that normally provokes pain.

Both hyperalgesia and allodynia describe psychophysical phenomena. Psychophysics is the study of the relationship between the physical world of objective external stimuli and the psychic world of internal subjective experiences of an organism. The experience of interest is of course pain, and how that might be related to quantifiable noxious stimuli. The discussion of these psychophysical terms here is limited to the context of verbal humans.

However, imprecise usage of these terms is commonly encountered in the pain world. In a philosophical handbook for pain medicine practice, it is important to discuss why the definitions above are unhelpful, if not also inappropriate. A divergence of perspective will be shown.

[3] It is again noted that the adjectives "nociceptive", "neuropathic" and "nociplastic" are hypotheses of mechanism of nociception, not descriptions of pain experience.

[4] Phenomenologically, (ii) includes (i) in the normal situation.

It will also be argued that the cardinal clinical sign of activation of a nociceptive apparatus is the phenomenon of allodynia, reconceptualised here as pain in response to a non-noxious stimulus. Examples of such stimuli include touch, pressure, distention or temperature variation, at intensities that do not cause tissue damage.

A Short History of Hyperalgesia

Historically, the two phenomena above were conflated by the pioneers in the investigative field of experimentally induced pain (technically, experimental engagement of nociception, EEN[5]), via the one term "hyperalgesia", which was first described as increased pain sensation due to either noxious or non-noxious stimulation of peripheral tissue (Willis 1992). In this initial denotation, the term did not imply any mechanism responsible for the phenomena.

Lewis and associates (Lewis 1942) were the first to report differences between the "hyperalgesia" localised to the area of cutaneous injury ("erythralgic hyperalgesia", p. 57) and the hyperalgesia found in adjacent non-injured skin ("diffuse hyperalgesia", p. 76). Hardy et al. (1950) introduced the terms "primary" and "secondary" hyperalgesia, to correspond respectively with Lewis' "erythralgic" and "diffuse" hyperalgesia.

This was the second connotation of the term "hyperalgesia", used to identify zones of increased sensitivity to stimuli, in damaged and undamaged tissue, induced by noxious stimulation of normal tissue.

"Primary hyperalgesia" (that is, the increased pain induced in the primary zone after experimental nociception) could be elicited by a thermal or a mechanical stimulus, leading to the terms "thermal hyperalgesia" and "mechanical hyperalgesia" respectively. This was shown to be attributable to sensitisation[6] of peripheral/primary nociceptors.[7]

This was the third connotation of the term "hyperalgesia", in which a mechanism is implied, irrespective of whether the inducing stimulus is noxious or innocuous.

Thus, there are three concurrent connotations of the one term, which has contributed to confusion in the literature:

(i) the blanket term of the phenomenon—no mechanism implied;
(ii) identification of zones following experimental nociception—an anatomical description; and,
(iii) when combined with a site-specific inducing stimulus—mechanism implied.

---

[5] Strictly, this field of investigation should be labelled "experimental engagement of nociception in order to examine behaviour considered to be analogous to the human pain experience". This leads to the acronym EEN, for experimental engagement of nociception, which will be used here.

[6] "Sensitisation" is relevant here only at the nerve fibre level and comprises (i) lowered threshold for discharge of fibre(s) of interest and/or (ii) increased firing of such fibre(s). This applies to peripheral and central neurons.

[7] There is an alternative, psychophysical, definition of hyperalgesia: leftward shift of the stimulus-response function that relates magnitude of pain to stimulus intensity (Ringkamp et al. 2013, p. 11).

Table 1 IASP definitions of hyperalgesia over time

Year	Source	Definition	Objection
1979	IASP Subcommittee on Taxonomy (Editorial, IASP 1979)	Increased sensitivity to noxious stimulation	"Sensitivity" undefined (See also chapter "Errors in Language and Logic Call for Epistemic Discipline")
1994	IASP 1994	Increased response to a stimulus which is normally painful (circular argument)	Stimuli are not "painful" (see chapter "Errors in Language and Logic Call for Epistemic Discipline") What is "normal"? Circular argument (see below)
2009	Recommended by IASP terminology committee	Increased response to a stimulus that is usually noxious	No objection: from a clinical point of view, this is correct
2011	Accepted by IASP Council	Increased pain from a stimulus that normally provokes pain	Reversion to 1994 definition

From the EEN perspective, connotation (iii) has evolved further, so that now the term "hyperalgesia" can be applied only to situations in which nociceptive afferents are involved.

Meanwhile, the official (IASP) definition of hyperalgesia has varied over time (Table 1).

It should be noted that to define HYPER-algesia as increased pain in response to "a stimulus that normally provokes pain" allows a back-derivation to NORMO-algesia—that is, pain—which then becomes defined as "pain from a stimulus that normally provokes pain", which is a circular argument. Furthermore, what is the baseline from which "increased pain" is to be determined? Or, to put that another way, how is a "normo-algesic" response to a noxious stimulus to be determined?[8]

It follows that the *only* definition of the phenomenon of hyperalgesia that is internally consistent with the current IASP lexicon is: *increased pain in response to a noxious stimulus*. However, this raises the ethical question of whether noxious stimuli should be used in the clinic.

A Short History of Allodynia

Historically, the concept of *allodynia* ("other pain") arose within the clinical perspective (as distinct from the EEN perspective), to denote pain induced by a non-noxious stimulus, especially in tissues that were ostensibly undamaged. However, that observation ran in parallel with the phenomenon of "secondary hyperalgesia" as identified in the EEN perspective, where non-injured skin adjacent to the area of induced nociception was found to be sensitive; namely, "pain behaviour" could be

[8] See also Cronje and Williamson (2006).

Table 2 IASP definitions of allodynia over time

Year.	Source	Definition	Objection
1979	IASP Subcommittee on taxonomy (Editorial, IASP 1979)	Pain due to a non-noxious stimulus to normal skin	Limited to "skin"
1994	IASP 1994	Pain due to a stimulus which does not normally provoke pain	What is "normal"? Circular argument (see below)
2009	Recommended by IASP terminology committee	Pain in response to a non-noxious stimulus	No objection: from a clinical point of view, this is correct
2011	Accepted by IASP Council	Pain due to a stimulus that does not normally provoke pain	Reversion to 1994 definition

elicited by a non-noxious stimulus applied to that area. This was shown to be mediated not by peripheral nociceptive afferents but rather by *non-nociceptive* afferents impinging on sensitised central nociceptive pathways (Ziegler et al. 1999).

Similarly to the case of hyperalgesia, the official (IASP) definition of allodynia has varied over time (Table 2).

To define allodynia in essence as pain in response to a stimulus that does not normally provoke pain again recapitulates that circular definition of "normoalgesia" as described above, as well as begging (that is, avoiding) the question of what is "normal".

It follows that the *only* definition of *clinical* allodynia that is internally consistent with the current IASP lexicon is: *pain in response to a non-noxious stimulus.*

Divergence of Perspectives

It can be seen that the confusion in the literature regarding the denotation and correct usage of the terms hyperalgesia and allodynia arises out of the differences between the EEN and clinical perspectives:

Perspective	Experimental nociception	Clinical
Focus	*Type of mediating nerve*	*Nature of stimulus*
Hyperalgesia	Nociceptive afferents	Noxious
Allodynia	Non-nociceptive afferents	Non-noxious

Currently, the only point of convergence of these perspectives is the elicitation of pain in normal tissue (clinical situation) or the secondary zone (EEN situation) in response to tangential stimulation of skin with a soft brush. This is always a non-noxious stimulus (satisfying clinical demands) that activates only non-nociceptive afferents (satisfying EEN demands) which, if it induces pain, allows the inference that central sensitisation of nociception may have occurred. This phenomenon has been labelled "dynamic cutaneous mechanical allodynia" or "brush allodynia".

This explanation may not account for pain induced in normal tissue by non-noxious pressure, whether punctate or blunt, or by non-noxious thermal stimuli or by non-noxious distention. Each of these is allodynia from a clinical perspective but has not yet been characterised from an EEN perspective.

The Interpretation of Allodynia in the Clinical Perspective

The phenomenon of clinical allodynia, as preferably defined as pain in response to a non-noxious stimulus, requires interpretation. The thesis here is that allodynia, whether spontaneously reported or specifically induced, is the fundamental clue to the state of activation of the nociceptive apparatus. In the current state of knowledge, the induction of pain by a non-noxious stimulus to normal tissue must imply that the nociceptive apparatus has been activated, probably at a central level, irrespective of which peripheral afferents can be shown to be involved. That latter important task remains with the EEN perspective, especially as it carries therapeutic potential.

The clinical recognition of nociplastic pain is a test case for this thesis. Although it is a decade since the construct of nociplastic pain was proposed (Chapter "The Salient Role of Nociception"), there is no consensus on how it may be recognised clinically in a formal sense. The essence of "nociplastic" is: not nociceptive, not neuropathic but nociception has been engaged.

In 2021, a set of diagnostic criteria for "chronic pain affecting the musculoskeletal system" was published (Kosek et al. 2021):

1. The pain is chronic, regional in distribution, and not explainable by a nociceptive or neuropathic process.
2. There is a history of pain hypersensitivity in the region of pain.
3. Presence of comorbidities:
   Any one of:
   (i) increased sensitivity to sound and/or light and/or odour,
   (ii) sleep disturbance with frequent nocturnal awakenings,
   (iii) fatigue,
   (iv) cognitive problems such as difficulty to focus attention, memory disturbances etc.
4. Evoked pain hypersensitivity phenomena can be elicited clinically in the region of pain.

A major objection to these criteria is the inclusion of the third set, the components of which are pathogenetically unrelated to nociception. It should be noted that neither "nociceptive" nor "neuropathic" nociception is identified by any criterion that is unrelated to nociception (Cohen 2022). This is an example of conflation of a hypothesis of mechanism (nociplastic) and clinical diagnosis ("typical" conditions), as discussed in chapter "The Salient Role of Nociception".

Despite the misnomer of "pain hypersensitivity" (see chapter "Errors in Language and Logic Call for Epistemic Discipline"), criterion 4—namely, allodynia—is the key feature that might allow inference of activation of a nociceptive apparatus.

A more appropriate approach would propose three criteria for the recognition of "nociplastic pain"[9]:

1. There is engagement of nociception which cannot be explained by a nociceptive or a neuropathic process.
2. Allodynia can be elicited clinically in the region of pain.
3. There is a history of hypersensitivity to non-noxious stimuli in the region of pain.

This area is currently being addressed by an IASP taskforce (Shraim et al. 2021; Shraim et al. 2026), a major confounding factor being ongoing conflation between nociplastic pain, clinical symptom clusters that may feature nociplastic pain, central sensitisation of nociception and primary pain (see chapter "The Salient Role of Nociception").

Therapeutic Implications

Many instances of chronic pain in humans are likely to be examples of persistent activation of the nociceptive apparatus (Middleton et al. 2021). Just how this occurs is the subject of intense research, complicated by the puzzle of why something that seems so maladaptive for humans has been so adaptive in an evolutionary sense.

The fundamental clinical expressions of sensitised nociception are spontaneous or persistent pain and pain in response to non-noxious stimuli, particularly touch, pressure and movement, that is, allodynia.

A therapeutic focus then would be to alleviate allodynia, as otherwise the organism may remain caught in a vicious (positive feedback) cycle. In the case of humans, the person needs to learn how to "protect" themself from the effects of persistent activation of the nociceptive apparatus and thus to reduce (or avoid) their pain experience.

---

[9] Technically, these criteria are for the recognition of nociplastic activation of a nociceptive apparatus, not "nociplastic pain".

So, how can clinical allodynia be alleviated? There are three main pathways, each of equal importance:

- Reducing the degree of nociception chemically, namely the prudent use of medication that might inhibit the transmission of nociceptive information to the brain in the first place (Sirucek et al. 2023), presuming that there is no ongoing "driver" of nociception.
- Limiting the degree of non-noxious stimulus that elicits allodynia, which translates into physically protecting the part; that is, not "pushing" outside the limits of tolerance (targeting "bottom-up" mechanisms).
- Trying to decrease nociception through cognitive approaches, which speaks to managing other stressors (targeting "top-down" mechanisms).

Detailed discussion of these pathways is beyond the scope of this Handbook.

Reducing Uncertainty

> It is imperative in science to doubt; it is absolutely necessary, for progress in science, to have uncertainty as a fundamental part of your inner nature. To make progress in understanding, we must remain modest and allow that we do not know. Nothing is certain or proved beyond all doubt. You investigate for curiosity, because it is unknown, not because you know the answer. (Feynman 2001: 247–248)

> Our value as physicians will lie in the gray-scale space, where we will have to support patients who are living with uncertainty — work that is essential to strong and meaningful doctor–patient relationships. (Simpkin and Schwartzstein 2016: 1714)

Confronting Uncertainty

Uncertainty describes "situations where knowledge or understanding is insufficient to allow for confident clinical decision making" (Tonelli and Upshur 2019:507). The patient's encounter with the *aporia* of pain (see chapter "Trying to Gain Traction on a Slippery Subject") compounds their discomfort with doubt about their own experience as well as how that might be seen by others. They present their body to the clinician for investigation and treatment with the quite reasonable expectation that the clinician will be able to explain their lived experience in scientific terms. The clinician encountering the *aporia* of the patient's experience may also be uncertain, uncomfortable and even dubious. Accepting uncertainty can be extremely difficult for clinicians because they share a "deeply rooted cultural unwillingness to acknowledge it" (Gheihmann et al. 2019:493). Thus, both parties are in the same position of lacking knowledge and understanding, which leads to a crisis of choice, of action and of identity (Burbules 2000). This uncertainty has potentially negative epistemic and moral implications for the therapeutic relationship (Cohen and Quintner 2012).

In chapter "The Clinical (Two-Person) Encounter" of this Handbook, it has been argued that this relationship—in the intersubjective space—is the most powerful vehicle for acknowledging this uncertainty and for negotiating towards validation. Four domains of intersubjectivity that might characterise the two-person encounter were identified: autonomy, shared humanity, empathy and trust. Two illustrative examples are given here of how this process towards validation can be perturbed.

Perturbation of Empathy: Stigmatisation

> Why is pain, something invisible and experienced by everyone—and therefore unlike the kinds of characteristics that usually lead to stigmatization—so often stigmatizing in its chronic form? (Jackson 2005: 332)

Stigmatisation has been defined as a process by which the reactions of a community to certain specific personal characteristics reduce a person's identity "from a whole and usual person to a tainted, discounted one", causing that person to be discredited, devalued, rejected and socially excluded from having a voice (Goffman 1963).

Examples of medically controversial—often termed "medically unexplained"—painful conditions that have been associated with stigmatisation of experiencers include "railway spine" and "occupation neurosis" in the nineteenth century (see chapter "Case Studies in Tautology, Circular Reasoning and Conflation: Fibromyalgia and Myofascial Pain "Syndromes""), and in the twentieth century, repetitive strain injury, "whiplash", non-specific low back pain and fibromyalgia. A common theme here has been to default to an inference of psychogenesis, in stark contrast to the relatively recently described neurobiological explanations for the clinical phenomena that characterise such conditions (Cohen et al. 2011).

The potential for stigmatisation in the clinic was mentioned in the discussion of application of Bourdieu's concepts in chapter "The Clinical (Two-Person) Encounter", specifically that of capital, with its inherent power imbalance. At the heart of stigmatisation of people experiencing pain is a unilateral, imposed and ostensibly "objective" interpretation of their predicament by health professionals. This precludes a reciprocal recognition and interpretation of stereotypes between the stigmatiser and the stigmatised "other" (Cohen et al. 2011).

This raises the question of whether stigmatisation may reflect a withdrawal of empathy by the clinician. Empathy implies a shared phenomenology wherein the observer is able to accept and understand the expression of another person's experience because it reflects that observer's own experience (Preston and de Waal 2002). It has been suggested that empathy functions as a foundation for other acts that allow one to live in the experience of the "other" in an intuitive manner, without needing to share that same experience especially at an emotional level (Stein 1917). Although commonly appreciated as a positive attribute (Gallagher 2006), empathy can embrace strong negative emotions, especially when the legitimacy of that person's distress is in doubt and their presentation challenges the observer's expectations and conceptual framing of the world. Empathy may then mutate into a projection of negative emotion and judgement toward the other person and even a conscious avoidance of compassion (Shaw et al. 1994).

For a clinician to recognise that their own behaviour may in fact be stigmatising can indeed be a challenge. Self-reflection invoking the domains of autonomy, shared humanity, empathy and trust, as described in chapter "The Clinical (Two-Person) Encounter", may be a useful approach.

Perturbation of Trust: Misinformation

Trust is recognised as being fundamental for the public understanding of science (Hendriks et al. 2016). In order to deal with scientific information, laypeople have to trust scientists and their findings. To the extent that clinical information should be scientifically based, such trust needs to be extended to clinicians.

This concept of trust has been expanded by Hendriks et al. (2016) as *epistemic trust*, which entails both assumption of dependence on the knowledge of others and vigilance toward the risk of being misinformed.

An example of violation of epistemic trust is the assertion that pain has a protective function:

> … pain has a protective role, and that persistent pain is often associated with substantially increased somatosensory stimulus-response profiles, consistent with an 'overprotective pain system'. (Ryan et al. 2024: 903)

Paraphrased, that statement states "The pain system has a protective role, which when overprotective can be associated with persistent pain". Apart from its internal contradiction (and the fiction of a "pain system"), this assertion raises two questions:

- against what is pain "protective"?
- how is pain "protective"?

Given that pain is contingent on nociception and that pain is an experience and not a concrete entity or "thing" with agentive properties (see chapter "Trying to Gain Traction on a Slippery Subject"), it follows firstly that it is nociception, not pain, that may have any "protective" function and, secondly, that any such function is to "protect" the organism from behaviour that may interfere with its recovery. In other words, *nociception protects the organism from itself.* In a chronic pain situation, it can be inferred that nociception is still engaged, even if there is no ongoing tissue damage. That engagement may in fact be central sensitisation of nociception.

This is not, as has been termed above, the manifestation of an "overprotective pain system" but rather the evolutionarily conserved function of a sensitised nociceptive apparatus that promotes the organism's survival (see chapter "Trying to Gain Traction on a Slippery Subject").

Therapeutic Possibilities for Reducing Uncertainty

> … the greatest comfort to a patient can be hearing that, regardless of clinical uncertainty, their physician will be with them no matter what the future brings. (Armstrong 2018:818)

Some of the contributory factors to uncertainty may be beyond influence, such as the answers to fundamental philosophical questions about pain. However, other contributors may well be amenable to alleviation, as are discussed in this Handbook:

- The inadequacy of the current (and former) IASP definitions of pain can be overcome by reformulation. (Chapter "Clarifying the Definition of Pain").
- Those problems of scientific language that are contingent upon pain-as-a-thing can be resolved through clarification. (Chapter "Errors in Language and Logic Call for Epistemic Discipline").
- The aphorism that nociception is necessary but not sufficient for pain, with the caveat that nociception be reconceptualised as activation of a nociceptive apparatus, is not only consistent with an evolutionary biological perspective but also has the potential to afford clinical, if not also societal and legal, legitimacy to many pain experiences that hitherto have been "medically unexplainable". (Chapter "The Salient Role of Nociception").
- A clear distinction can be made between pain, suffering and pain-related suffering. Not all pain experiences are necessarily associated with suffering and not all suffering in a person experiencing pain may be due to nociception. (Chapter "Trying to Gain Traction on a Slippery Subject").
- Understanding the intersubjectivity that defines the clinical encounter, through the avenues of autonomy, shared humanity, empathy and trust, can facilitate communication between patient and health care professional towards *mutual* benefit. (Chapter "The Clinical (Two-Person) Encounter").

More broadly, that nociception is not sufficient for pain speaks to those non-nociception-related factors that are the "bridge" between that process and the pain experience. These may well lie in the "black box" that constitutes the "person", being underpinned by the complex function of the central nervous system, especially the brain and, ultimately, the phenomenon of consciousness. This then refers to the psychological ("-psycho-") dimension of the frameworks discussed in chapters "Conceptual Frameworks" and "The Clinical (Two-Person) Encounter". These factors, which have not been addressed in any detail here but may well mediate the "top-down" influences on activation of the nociceptive apparatus, are to be found in the patient's history, especially that which relates to exposure to stressors, whether somatic, psychological or environmental. When mutual trust has been established within a therapeutic relationship, the word "comfort" can be employed in its original meaning, "to give strength and hope to a person".[10]

Diagnostic Formulation

> All these problems illustrate the central role of diagnosis itself. Perhaps most fundamentally, the act of diagnosis links the individual to the social system; it is necessarily a spectacle as well as a bureaucratic event. Diagnosis remains a ritual of disclosure: a curtain is pulled aside, and uncertainty is replaced—for better or worse—by a structured narrative. (Rosenberg 2002, p. 255)

Medical diagnoses tend to be concrete concepts, simultaneously implying understanding of a condition and the therapeutic pathway to be followed. Diagnosis (from the Greek: *dia* denoting "through" and *gnosis* denoting "knowledge") originally referred to the process of identifying, in the body, underlying causes and associations considered to be responsible for the patient's complaints and then conferring a label (also called "diagnosis"). Such labels have come to imply deeper inherent knowledge, if not also certainty, which is often difficult to justify in the context of pain.

In the clinic, with its intrinsic purposes of diagnosis, explanation and management of a patient's predicament, capturing that complexity comprehensively and concisely poses a major challenge. To date, pain medicine has struggled with language and nomenclature: the words that are used and the concepts they entail are fluid and imprecise, in a situation where the clinical situation demands the opposite.

This challenge can be met by moving away from the conventional process of "diagnosis" towards one of formulation of the predicament that the patient is facing. Clinical formulations also have important social implications, including providing a working language for health planners, employers, lawyers and insurers, influencing healthcare and disability payments and conferring exemption from social responsibilities. A multifactorial clinical problem such as pain requires a multiaxial conceptual framework in order to develop both a working understanding of and a therapeutic approach to the individual patient's predicament.

What is presented here is an approach to formulation, both as a process and as a working document intended for diagnostic and therapeutic purposes and for communication. Some of this material is also to be found in the training document *Clinical Formulation in Pain Medicine* of the Faculty of Pain Medicine, Australian and New Zealand College of Anaesthetists,[11] to which the authors contributed, and used here with permission.

---

[10] www.merriam-webster.com/dictionary/comfort

[11] www.fpm.anzca.edu.au

The Concept of Multiaxial Formulation

The practice of multiaxial formulation was first developed in psychiatry, and arose naturally from child psychiatry, where functioning and contextual factors had always been recognised as important in management. The term "multiaxial diagnosis" was coined by the English child and family psychiatrist Michael Rutter (1975). In 1980, the third edition of the *Comprehensive Textbook of Psychiatry* (Kaplan et al. 1980) promoted the three central domains: diagnosis, functioning and context. This evolved, via the WHO 1997 publication "Multiaxial Presentation of the ICD 10 for use in Adult Psychiatry", into the International Classification of Functioning Disability and Health WHO 2001 (ICF).

The multiaxial matrix outlined here is an integration of two frameworks:

- The *dimensions* of the biopsychosocial (or sociopsychobiomedical) paradigm, as discussed in chapter "Conceptual Frameworks":

Bio-	What's happening to the person's body?
-psycho-	What's happening to the person?
-social	What's happening in the person's world?

and

- The *domains* of the International Classification of Functioning Disability and Health (ICF, WHO 2001):

Diagnosis	What is the matter?
Functioning and disability	How bad is it?
Context	Personal and environmental factors

What Is the Matter?

This domain is the conventional list of diagnoses, medical and psychiatric. The recent inclusion of pain as a condition-in-its-own-right in ICD-11 (see chapter "The Non-Convergent Language Used in Clinical and Taxonomic Settings") and the evolving area of "pain descriptors"—technically, hypotheses of mechanism of nociception (see chapter "The Salient Role of Nociception")—offer the possibility of more nuanced somatic diagnostic labels, as will be discussed under Nomenclature below.

How "Bad" Is it?

Assessment of functioning and disability is described under the three sub-domains below that correspond to the older WHO concepts of impairment, disability and handicap, but expressed in less discriminatory language:

- Function—effect on functioning at the level of the *organ or system.*
- Activity—effect on functioning at the level of the *organism*, the ability to do things, such as walking, sitting, standing, lifting, carrying.
- Participation—effect on *interpersonal* functioning, in the family, at work, in social life.

Context: Personal and Environmental Factors

Context refers to any personal or environmental factor that will alter the course of the condition, for better or for worse. Contextual factors provide opportunities for treatment and insights about prognosis that do not naturally arise from diagnosis or associated functional factors.

In the assessment matrix below, which attempts to present the dimensions of the biopsychosocial (or sociopsychobiomedical) framework and the domains of ICF in two axes, a non-exhaustive list of contextual factors is offered. This matrix is an example of a heuristic for the clinician to organise complex information into a coherent whole and, in particular, to identify where and what type of therapeutic interventions may be appropriate. In any one clinical case, not all the cells need to have entries (Table 3).

Towards a New Nomenclature for Clinical Pain Problems

The Inadequacy of Current Nomenclature

Conventional diagnostic labels for most pain conditions have either incorporated the symptom "pain" into a pseudo-diagnosis, such as "low back pain" or "pain syndrome", or have used suffixes taken from Greek words for pain, such as "neur-*algia*" or "coccy-*dynia*". In effect, these labels are not only confined to the somatic dimension but also tend to imply that the anatomical structure(s) or region(s) in which the pain is experienced is also the origin of nociception.

Table 3 A clinical assessment matrix

		DOMAINS		
		Diagnosis What is the matter?	Functioning How bad is it?	Context Personal and environmental factors
DIMENSIONS	BIO-What's happening to the person's body?	*Somatic* Conventional labels Hypothesis of nociception label	Effect on bodily function and structure	Medication
	-PSYCHO- What's happening to the person?	*Psychological/psychiatric* DSM-5 labels	Effect on whole-person activities	Behaviours and strategies Beliefs and understanding Development and education Emotions
	-SOCIAL What's happening in the person's world?	Housing, social and economic circumstances Employment status	Effect on participation	Education and literacy Family history of diseases or disabilities Lifestyle and life management issues Negative events in childhood Primary support group including family Legal issues

A number of relatively recent developments discussed in this Handbook have highlighted the inadequacy of such conventional labels. Firstly, the advent of bio-psychosocial frameworks for facilitating a whole-person understanding of the pain experience demands that language be found to describe the psychological and social dimensions. Secondly, the choice of words in the paragraph immediately above of "origin of nociception" instead of "where the pain is coming from" highlights the all-important distinction to be made between those two phenomena.

Thirdly, as a fundamental principle, "pain" cannot be used as a clinical diagnostic term for any condition in which "pain" is a symptom. However, this admonition runs contrary to a recent development in the epistemology of pain, namely the *taxonomic* recognition of pain as a condition-in-its-own-right as incorporated into ICD-11 (see chapter "The Non-Convergent Language Used in Clinical and Taxonomic Settings"). This implies that pain is a "thing" (see chapter "Trying to Gain Traction on a Slippery Subject") and thus might justify the use of the word as a clinical diagnosis.

In ICD-11, (chronic) pain is classified as "secondary" if the experience occurs in the context of an identifiable disease or damage state. That means that an anatomical origin of nociception can be identified, more or less confidently, and that a mechanism of nociception can be inferred. Such a mechanism is limited to "nociceptive" or "neuropathic" in ICD-11 (see chapter "The Salient Role of Nociception").

By contrast, if chronic pain "... cannot be better accounted for by another chronic pain condition" (Treede et al. 2015), then it is classified in ICD-11 as "primary". This implies that neither an origin nor a mechanism of nociception can confidently be found.

In parallel with this, a fourth development has emerged, namely the construct of "nociplastic pain", defined essentially as pain that is not associated with nociceptive or neuropathic mechanisms of nociception but is associated with clinical features suggesting that nociception has nonetheless been engaged.

As discussed in chapter "The Salient Role of Nociception", in the current state of play, there has been conflation between primary pain and nociplastic pain, a situation partly attributable to the current lack of validated clinical criteria for identifying the latter. Of course, once "nociplastic pain" has been validated, then the pain of conditions that are found to feature this will move out of the "primary" into the "secondary" category. Neither "primary" nor "secondary" carries any insight into the mechanism of nociception underlying the pain.

For this reason alone, an argument can be made that the ICD-11 categories should not be used for clinical diagnoses. Instead, the descriptors of nociception—nociceptive, neuropathic and nociplastic—could be invoked as part of a clinical diagnostic label.

An Approach to a New Nomenclature for Clinical Pain Conditions

An optimal system of nomenclature for clinical pain conditions should capture succinctly the three dimensions of a biopsychosocial (or sociopsychobiomedical) conceptual framework.

As has been discussed in this Handbook, nociception (in the "bio" or "biomedical" dimension) is the necessary pre-condition for pain (Weisman et al. 2026). It follows that, without denying their influence on modifying the pain experience and therefore their importance in clinical formulation, none of the factors listed in the psychological or social dimensions in Table 3 is necessary or sufficient for a pain experience.

Therefore, it is of prime importance that nomenclature for the somatic (or biomedical) *dimension* or, if preferred, the diagnosis *domain* (see previous section) convey as much information as possible about both the state of activation of the nociceptive apparatus and any underlying disease or noxious process. It is also recognised that it is this dimension or domain that determines coding for epidemiological, administrative and remunerative purposes.

Such a nomenclature needs to reflect two current issues. Firstly, it is well recognised by clinicians that the mere presence of a structural abnormality (such as osteoarthrosis or spondylosis) neither predicts that pain in the region will be experienced nor justifies an inference that it is a site of nociception responsible for a complaint of pain (Chou et al. 2012; de Schepper et al. 2010). Second is the trend towards clinically identifying mechanisms of nociception, both known (nociceptive and neuropathic) and hypothesised (nociplastic) (Shraim et al. 2021; Shraim et al. 2026).

For instance, to label a problem of pain in the knee as "(osteo)arthritis of the knee" or to attribute pain in the back to "spondylosis" is both inaccurate and inadequate.

Therefore, a somatic diagnostic dyad is suggested, that consists of

(i) mechanism of activation of the nociceptive apparatus—MANA; and
(ii) underlying pathological/pathophysiological process (if identified)—UPP (Table 4).

Capturing the "Psychological" and "Social" Dimensions in a Diagnostic Label

This discussion addresses only the top left-hand cell of the assessment matrix presented above. Application of DSM-5 (American Psychiatric Association 2013) labels to the clinical pain situation is an exercise that is beyond the scope of this Handbook. However, the other seven cells in the matrix can be used as a heuristic for constructing a narrative summary of the patient's predicament in the psychological ("whole person") and social ("person's world") dimensions.

Table 4 Examples of application of a somatic diagnostic dyad

Clinical scenario	Conventional label	Somatic diagnostic dyad	
		MANA	UPP
Knee pain where structural abnormality is known	Osteoarthritis	Nociceptive (activation of mechanonociceptors)	Osteoarthrosis
Knee pain in context of, say, rheumatoid arthritis	Rheumatoid arthritis	Nociceptive (inflammation)	Inflammatory arthropathy
Pain in an apparently structurally normal knee	"Knee pain"	Nociceptive OR nociplastic	Possible biomechanical dysfunction of the knee OR region of somatic referred pain
Pain ± paraesthesiae ± motor dysfunction in the hand	"Carpal tunnel syndrome"	Neuropathic	Compression neuropathy of the median nerve in the carpal tunnel
Pain + allodynia post *herpes zoster* infection	"Post-herpetic neuralgia"	Neuropathic	Post-*herpes zoster* neuropathy (dorsal root ganglion dysfunction)
Painful diabetic neuropathy	Diabetic peripheral neuropathy	Neuropathic	Diabetic peripheral neuropathy
Pain ± allodynia ± vasomotor changes in the arm	Complex regional pain syndrome	Nociplastic	Regional upper limb impairment
Chronic widespread pain	"Fibromyalgia"	Nociplastic	Impairment of (site of pain)
Chronic low back pain	"Chronic low back pain"	Nociceptive or nociplastic	Lumbar spondylosis and/or biomechanical dysfunction of the lumbar spine
Leg pain in segmental distribution + signs of radiculopathy	"Sciatica" (obsolete)	Neuropathic	Lumbar radiculopathy
Leg pain in non-segmental distribution with no signs of neurological deficit		Nociplastic	Region of somatic referred pain

References

American Psychiatric Association. DSM-5 task force. Diagnostic and statistical manual of mental disorders: DSM-5™. 5th ed. American Psychiatric Publishing Inc.; 2013. https://doi.org/10.1176/appi.books.9780890425596.

Armstrong K. If you can't beat it, join it: uncertainty and trust in medicine. Ann Int Med. 2018;168(11):818–9. https://doi.org/10.7326/M18-0445.

Burbules NC. Aporias, webs and passages: doubt as an opportunity to learn. Curric Inq. 2000;30:171–87. https://doi.org/10.1111/0362-6784.00161.

Chou R, Deyo RA, Jarvik JG. Appropriate use of lumbar imaging for evaluation of low back pain. Radiol Clin. 2012;50(4):569–85. https://doi.org/10.1016/j.rcl.2012.04.005.

Cohen ML. The proposed clinical criteria for nociplastic pain in the musculoskeletal system are flawed. Pain. 2022;163:e606–7. https://doi.org/10.1097/j.pain.0000000000002505.

Cohen ML, Quintner JL. The clinical conversation about pain: tensions between the lived experience and the biomedical model. In: McKenzie H, Quintner JL, Bendelow G, editors. At the edge of being: the aporia of pain. Oxford: Interdisciplinary Press; 2012. p. 19–35.

Cohen ML, Quintner JL, Buchanan D, Nielsen M, Guy L. Stigmatization of patients with chronic pain: the extinction of empathy. Pain Med. 2011;12:1637–43. https://doi.org/10.1111/j.1526-4637.2011.01264.x.

Cronje RJ, Williamson OD. Is pain ever "normal"? Clin J Pain. 2006;22:92–699. https://doi.org/10.1097/01.ajp.0000210919.03289.1e.

de Schepper EI, Damen J, van Meurs JB, Ginai AZ, Popham M, Hofman A, Koes BW, Bierma-Zeinstra SM. The association between lumbar disc degeneration and low back pain: the influence of age, gender, and individual radiographic features. Spine. 2010;35(5):531–6. https://doi.org/10.1097/BRS.0b013e3181aa5b33.

Editorial. The need of a taxonomy. Pain. 1979;6(3):247–52. https://doi.org/10.1016/0304-3959(79)90046-0.

Feynman R. The pleasure of finding things out: the best short works of Richard Feynman. London: Penguin Books; 2001.

Gallagher RM. Empathy: a timeless skill for the pain medicine toolbox. Pain Med. 2006;7:213–4. https://doi.org/10.1111/j.1526-4637.2006.00163.x.

Gheihmann G, Johnson M, Simpkin AL. Twelve tips for thriving in the face of clinical uncertainty. Med Teach. 2019;42(5):493–9. https://doi.org/10.1080/014219X.2019.1579308.

Goffman E. Stigma: notes on the management of spoiled identity. New York: Prentice Hall; 1963.

Hardy JD, Wolff HG, Goodell H. Experimental evidence on the nature of cutaneous hyperalgesia. J Clin Invest. 1950;29(1):115–40.

Hendriks F, Kienhues D, Bromme R. Trust in science and the science of trust. In: Blöbaum B, editor. Trust and communication in a digitized world: models and concepts of trust research. Cham: Springer; 2016. p. 143–59. https://doi.org/10.1007/978-3-319-28059-2_8.

Jackson JE. Stigma, liminality, and chronic pain. Am Ethnol. 2005;32:332–53. https://doi.org/10.1525/ae.2005.32.3.332.

Kaplan H, Freedman AM, Sadock BJ, editors. Comprehensive textbook of psychiatry III. William and Wilkins: Philadephia; 1980.

Kosek E, Clauw D, Nijs J, Baron R, Gilron I, Harris RE, Mico J-A, Rice ASC, Sterling M. Chronic nociplastic pain affecting the musculoskeletal system: clinical criteria and grading system. Pain. 2021;162:2629–34. https://doi.org/10.1097/j.pain.0000000000002324.

Lewis T. Pain. New York: The Macmillan Company; 1942.

Middleton SJ, Barry AM, Comini M, Li Y, Ray PR, Shiers S, et al. Studying human nociceptors: from fundamentals to clinic. Brain. 2021;144:1312–35. https://doi.org/10.1093/brain/awab048.

Preston SD, de Waal FBM. Empathy: its ultimate and proximate bases. Behav Brain Sci. 2002;25:1–72. https://doi.org/10.1017/s0140525x02000018.

Ringkamp M, Raja SN, Campbell JN, Meyer RA. Peripheral mechanisms of cutaneous nociception. In: McMahon SB, Koltzenberg M, Tracy I, Turk D, editors. Wall and Melzack's textbook of pain. 6th ed. Philadelphia: Elsevier; 2013. p. 1–30.

Rosenberg CE. The tyranny of diagnosis: specific entities and individual experience. Milbank Q. 2002;80(2):237–60. https://doi.org/10.1111/1468-0009.t01-1-00003.

Rutter M, Shaffer D, Shepherd M, World Health Organization. In: Shaffer D, Shepherd M, editors. A multi-axial classification of child psychiatric disorders: an evaluation of a proposal/Michael Rutter. Geneva: World Health Organization; 1975.

Ryan CG, Karran EL, Wallwork SB, Pate JW, O'Keefe M, Fullen BM, Livadas N, Jones N, Toumbourou JW, Gilchrist P, Cameron PA, Fatoye F, Ravindran D, Moseley GL. We are all in this together—whole of community pain science education campaign to promote better management of persistent pain. J Pain. 2024;25(4):902–17. https://doi.org/10.1016/j.jpain.2023.10.024.

Shaw LL, Batson CD, Todd RM. Empathy avoidance: forestalling feeling for another in order to escape the motivational consequences. J Pers Soc Psychol. 1994;67:879–87.

Shraim MA, Massé-Alarie H, Hodges PW. Methods to discriminate between mechanism-based categories of pain experienced in the musculoskeletal system: a systematic review. Pain. 2021;162(4):1007–37. https://doi.org/10.1097/j.pain.0000000000002113.

Shraim MA, Sterling M, Sluka KA, Arendt-Nielsen L, Backonja M, Baron R, Blechschmidt V, Clauw DJ, Cohen M, Coombes BK, Elsenbruch S, Gilron I, Harris RE, Jones LE, Kapreli E, Kato F, Kosek E, Madden VJ, Nijs J, Reis FJJ, Rice AC, Ringkamp M, Schmid AB, Irani A, Veasle C, Hodges PW. Towards a tool to discriminate between pain mechanistic descriptors: expert ranking of features and allocation of weights using a forced choice paradigm. Pain., in press. 2026;

Simpkin AL, Schwartzstein RM. Tolerating uncertainty—the next medical revolution? N Engl J Med. 2016;375:1713–5. https://doi.org/10.1056/NEJMp1606402.

Sirucek L, Ganley RP, Zeilhofer HU, Schweinhardt P. Diffuse noxious inhibitory controls and conditioned pain modulation: a shared neurobiology within the descending pain inhibitory system? Pain. 2023;164(3):463–8. https://doi.org/10.1097/j.pain.0000000000002719.

Stein E. On the problem of empathy. Stein W, trans. Washington, DC: ICS Publications; 1917.

Tonelli MR, Upshur REG. A philosophical approach to addressing *uncertainty* in medical education. Acad Med. 2019;94:507–11. https://doi.org/10.1097/ACM.0000000000002512.

Treede R-D, Rief W, Barke A, Aziz Q, Bennett MI, Benoliel R, Cohen M, Evers S, Finnerup NB, First MB, Giamberardino MA, Kaasa S, Kosek E, Lavand'homme P, Nicholas M, Perrot S, Scholz J, Schug S, Smith BH, Svensson P, Vlaeyen JWS, Wang S-J. A classification of chronic pain for ICD-11. Pain. 2015;156:1003–7. https://doi.org/10.1097/j.pain.00000000.

Weisman A, Quintner J, Cohen M. Adieu to an aphorism: nociception is necessary for pain. Brain. 2026;149(2):422–31. https://doi.org/10.1093/brain/awaf387.

WHO. International classification of functioning, disability, and health: ICF. Geneva: World Health Organization; 2001.

Willis WD. Hyperalgesia and allodynia: summary and overview. In: Willis W, editor. Hyperalgesia and allodynia. New York: Raven Press; 1992. p. 1–11.

Ziegler EA, Magerl W, Meyer RA, Treede R-D. Secondary hyperalgesia to punctate mechanical stimuli: central sensitization to A-fibre nociceptive input. Brain. 1999;122(12):2245–57. https://doi.org/10.1093/brain/122.12.2245.

Appendix: Joint Peer-Reviewed Publications by the Authors

Book Chapters

1. Cohen ML, Quintner JL. The clinical conversation about pain: tensions between the lived experience and the biomedical model. In: Fernandez J, editor. Making Sense of Pain: Critical and Interdisciplinary Perspectives. Oxford: Interdisciplinary Press; 2010a: pp. 85–100. [ISBN: 978-1-84888-36-8] http://www.inter-disciplinary.net/publishing/id-press/ebooks/making-sense-of-pain/.
2. Cohen ML, Quintner JL. The clinical conversation about pain: tensions between the lived experience and the biomedical model. Part 1. Complexities of Pain. In: Quintner J, McKenzie H, Bendelow G, editors. At the Edge of Being: the Aporia of Pain. Oxford: Interdisciplinary Press; 2010b: pp. 19–35. [ISBN: 978-90-04-39922-8] http://interdisciplinarypress.net/online-store/medical-humanities/at-the-edge-of-being-the-aporia-of-pain. https://doi.org/10.1163/9781848880368_009.
3. Quintner JL, Cohen ML. Myofascial pain—a failed construct. Chapter 14 In: Hutson M, Ward A, editors. Oxford Textbook of Musculoskeletal Medicine, 2nd ed. Oxford: Oxford University Press; 2016a: pp. 132–142 [ISBN 978-0-19-967410-7].
4. Cohen ML, Quintner JL. Pain concepts – chronic pain. Chapter 19 In: Hutson M, Ward A, editors. Oxford Textbook of Musculoskeletal Medicine. 2nd ed. Oxford: Oxford University Press; 2016: pp. 179–185. [ISBN 978-0-19-967410-7].
5. Quintner JL, Cohen ML. The challenge of validating the experience of chronic pain: the importance of intersubjectivity and reframing In: Van Rysewyk S, editor. Human Meanings of Pain. Springer, Cham; 2016b. pp. 281–293. ISBN Reference: 978-3-319-49022-9. https://doi.org/10.1007/978-3-319-49022-9_17.
6. Cohen ML, Quintner JL. Is "chronic pain" a meaningful diagnosis? Chapter 13 In: Van Rysewyk S, ed. Human Meanings of Pain, vol. 2. Cham: Springer Verlag, 2019: pp. 249–260. [ISBN 978-3-030-24153-7] https://link.springer.com/book/10.1007%2F978-3-030-24154-4.

M. Cohen, J. Quintner, *A Philosophical Handbook for Pain Medicine Practice*,
https://doi.org/10.1007/978-981-92-1682-6

7. Quintner JL, Galbraith M, Cohen ML. Connotations of pain in a socio-psycho-biological framework. Chapter 12 In: Van Rysewyk S, editor. Human Meanings of Pain, vol 2. Cham: Springer Verlag, 2019: pp. 233–248. [ISBN 978-3-030-24153-7] https://link.springer.com/book/10.1007%2F978-3-030-24154-4

Refereed Journal Publications

1. Cohen ML, Quintner JL. Fibromyalgia syndrome, a problem of tautology. Lancet. 1993;342:904–908. https://doi.org/10.1016/0140-6736(93)91950-Q
2. Quintner JL, Cohen ML. Referred pain of peripheral neural origin: an alternative to the "myofascial pain" construct. Clin J Pain. 1994a;10:243–251. https://doi.org/10.1097/00002508-199409000-00012.
3. Quintner JL, Cohen ML. Occupation neuroses and the psychogenic connotation of "repetition strain injury": the misconstruction of neurosis. Integ Psychiatr. 1994b;10:165–176.
4. Cohen ML, Quintner JL. The derailment of "railway spine": a timely lesson for post-traumatic fibromyalgia. Pain Rev. 1996;3:181–202.
5. Cohen ML, Quintner JL. Fibromyalgia syndrome and disability: a failed construct fails those in pain. Med J Aust. 1998;168:402–404. PMID: 9594952.
6. Quintner JL, Cohen ML. Fibromyalgia falls foul of a fallacy. Lancet. 1999;353:1092–1094. https://doi.org/10.1016/S0140-6736(98)06468-X
7. Quintner JL, Buchanan D, Cohen ML, Taylor A. Signification and pain: a semiotic reading of fibromyalgia. Theor Med. 2003;24:345–354. https://doi.org/10.1023/A:1026061420192
8. Quintner JL, Cohen ML, Buchanan D, Katz J, Williamson OW. Pain medicine and its models: helping or hindering? Pain Med. 2008;9:824–834. https://doi.org/10.1111/j.1526-4637.2007.00391.x
9. Lyon P, Cohen ML, Quintner JL. An evolutionary stress-response hypothesis for chronic widespread pain (fibromyalgia syndrome). Pain Med. 2011;12:1167–1178. https://doi.org/10.1111/j.1526-4637.2011.01168.x
10. Cohen M, Quintner J, Buchanan D, Nielsen A, Guy L. Stigmatization of patients with chronic pain: the extinction of empathy. Pain Med. 2011;12:1637–1643. https://doi.org/10.1111/j.1526-4637.2011.01264.x
11. Cohen ML, Quintner J, Buchanan D. Is chronic pain a disease? Pain Med. 2013;14:1284–1288. https://doi.org/10.1111/pme.12025
12. Quintner JL, Bove GM, Cohen ML. A critical evaluation of the trigger point phenomenon. Rheumatology. 2015;54:392–399. https://doi.org/10.1093/rheumatology/keu471.
13. Cohen ML, Quintner JL, Van Rysewyk S. Reconsidering the IASP definition of pain. Pain Rep. 2018;3(e634):1–7. https://doi.org/10.1097/PR9.0000000000000634.

14. Cohen M, Weisman A, Quintner J. Pain is not a "thing": how that error affects language and logic in pain medicine. J Pain. 2022;23(8):1283–1293. https://doi.org/10.1016/j.jpain.2022.03.235.
15. Cohen M, Quintner J, Weisman A. "Nociplastic" pain: a challenge to nosology and to nociception. J Pain. 2023;24:2131–2139. https://doi.org/10.1016/j.pain.2023.07.019.
16. Cohen ML, Weisman A, Quintner JL. Paradoxes weaken the IASP definition of pain. Korean J Pain. 2026;39(1):51–58. https://doi.org/10.3344/kjp.25268.
17. Weisman A, Quintner J, Cohen M. Adieu to an aphorism: why nociception *is* necessary for pain. Brain. 2026;149:422–431. https://doi.org/10.1093/brain/awaf387.

Other Contributions to Peer-Reviewed Journals (Editorials; Letters)

1. Quintner JL, Cohen ML. Soft tissue rheumatism. [Letter] Mod Med Aust. 1993;157:358.
2. Champion GD, Cohen ML, Quintner JL. Fibromyalgia in the workplace. [Letter] Ann Rheum Dis. 1993;52:836–837.
3. Quintner JL, Cohen ML. The fibromyalgia controversy. [Letter] Mod Med Aust. 1995;38(9):17.
4. Cohen ML, Quintner JL. Comment on "fibromyalgia" (pain 60 (1995) 349–350). [Letter] Pain. 1996;64:393.
5. Cohen ML, Quintner JL. Response to Hadler "Carpal Tunnel Syndrome: diagnostic conundrum.". [Letter] J Rheumatol. 1997;24:2485.
6. Quintner JL, Cohen ML. Fibromyalgia syndrome. [Letter] Med J Aust. 1997;166:168.
7. Cohen ML, Quintner JL. Altered nociception but not fibromyalgia after cervical spine injury: comment on the article by Buskila et al. [Letter] Arthritis Rheum. 1998;41:183.
8. Quintner JL, Cohen ML. Comment on Focus article by Aronoff and commentaries: 'Myofascial pain syndrome and fibromyalgia: a critical assessment and alternate view'. [Letter] Clin J Pain. 1999;15:155–157.
9. Cohen ML, Quintner JL. Comment on Pain elicited by blunt pressure: neurobiological basis and clinical relevance. Treede et al (Pain 98 (2002) 235). [Letter] Pain 2003;104:711–716.
10. Quintner JL, Cohen ML. Economic cost and epidemiological characteristics of fibromyalgia syndrome. [Letter] J Rheumatol. 2004;31:2311.
11. Williamson OD, Buchanan DA, Quintner JL, Cohen ML. Pain beyond monism and dualism. [Letter] Pain. 2005;116:169–170.

12. Cohen ML, Quintner JL. Comment on Vierck CJ Jr: Mechanisms underlying development of spatially distributed chronic pain (fibromyalgia). [Letter] Pain. 2007;129:224–226.
13. Cohen ML, Quintner JL. The horse is dead: let myofascial pain syndrome rest in peace. [Letter]. Pain Med. 2008;9:464–465.
14. Quintner JL, Buchanan D, Cohen ML. Maldynia as a moral judgement. [Letter] Pain Med. 2011;12:1130.
15. Cohen M, Quintner J, Buchanan D, Nielsen A, Guy L. Response to letter from Dr Mark Awerbuch regarding Pain Medicine 2011;12:1637–1643. [Letter] Pain Med. 2012;13:1092–1093.
16. Quintner JL, Cohen ML. Are peripheral pain generators important in fibromyalgia and chronic widespread pain? [Letter] Pain Med. 2014;15:718–719.
17. Quintner JL, Cohen ML. Myofascial trigger points in patients with whiplash-associated disorders and mechanical neck pain. [Letter] Pain Med. 2015;16:828–629.
18. Quintner JL, Bove GM, Cohen ML. Response to Dommerholt and Gerwin: did we miss the point? [Letter] J Bodyw Mov Ther. 2015a;19(3):394–395.
19. Quintner JL, Bove GM, Cohen ML. Comment on a critical evaluation of the trigger point phenomenon. [Letter] Rheumatology. 2015b;54:1127–1128.
20. Van Rysewyk S, Quintner J, Galbraith M, Cohen M. Do we mean to ignore meaning in pain? [Editorial] Pain Med. 2021;22(5):1021–1023.
21. Quintner JL, Cohen ML. A new definition of pain: update and implications for physical therapy practice and rehabilitation science. [Letter] Phys Ther J. 2021;101(9):pzab136.
22. Weisman A, Quintner J, Cohen M, Maharawi Y. Commentary on "central sensitisation in chronic pain conditions: latest discoveries and their potential for precision medicine". [Letter] Lancet Rheumatol. 2021;3:e547.
23. Cohen M, Weisman A, Quintner J. Response to van Rysewyk S and Moseley GL et al.'s comments on Cohen et al. J Pain 2022;23(8):1283–1293. [Letter] J Pain. 2023;24:184–185.
24. Weisman A, Quintner J, Cohen M. "Primary" versus "secondary" musculoskeletal pain: the pitfall of dichotomy. [Letter] J Pain. 2024;25(11):104510.
25. Cohen M, Weisman A, Quintner J. Contesting the BACPAP Consortium's consensus. [Letter] Lancet Rheumatol. 2024;6(7):e419.
26. Quintner J, Weisman A, Cohen M. Nociplastic pain: controversy of the concept. [Letter] Korean J Pain. 2025;38(2):213–214.
27. Cohen M, Quintner J, Weisman A. "Primary" and "nociplastic" pain must not be conflated. [Letter] Pain. 2025;156:1949–1950.
28. Cohen M, Quintner J, Weisman A. Conflations compound nociplastic pain. [Letter] Pain. 2026a; 167:1240–1241.
29. Cohen ML, Quintner JL, Weisman A. Defining the boundary between pain and suffering. [Letter] Pain. 2026b; 167(7):1730–1731.

GPSR Compliance

The European Union's (EU) General Product Safety Regulation (GPSR) is a set of rules that requires consumer products to be safe and our obligations to ensure this.

If you have any concerns about our products, you can contact us on ProductSafety@springernature.com

In case Publisher is established outside the EU, the EU authorized representative is:

Springer Nature Customer Service Center GmbH
Europaplatz 3
69115 Heidelberg, Germany

Batch number: 10889560

Printed by Printforce, the Netherlands